VIVA VOCE, MODEL QUESTIONS and QUESTION BANK

for

Diploma and Degree Courses in

PHARMACY

Section A

VIVA VOCE QUESTIONS

Including Practical-Oriented Questions

Section B

MODEL QUESTIONS

Based on Board Examination Papers

Section C

QUESTION BANK

Selected Questions of Paper-Setters' Choice

VIVA VOCE, MODEL QUESTIONS and QUESTION BANK

for

Diploma and Degree Courses in PHARMACY

R. Raveendra

Professor
R.R. College of Pharmacy
Bangalore 560090
Former Principal
Raman College of Pharmacy
Bangalore 560086

CBS

CBS Publishers & Distributors Pvt. Ltd.

New Delhi • Bengaluru • Chennai • Kochi • Kolkata • Mumbai
Hyderabad • Uttarakhand • Nagpur • Patna • Pune • Jharkhand

ISBN: 81-239-1484-9

First Edition: 2007
Reprint: 2007, 2015, 2018, 2019

Published by **Satish Kumar Jain** and produced by **Varun Jain** for
CBS Publishers & Distributors Pvt. Ltd.,
4819/XI Prahlad Street, 24 Ansari Road, Daryaganj, New Delhi - 110002
delhi@cbspd.com, cbspubs@airtelmail.in • www.cbspd.com
Ph.: 23289259, 23266861, 23266867 • Fax: 011-23243014

Corporate Office: 204 FIE, Industrial Area, Patparganj, Delhi - 110 092
Ph: 49344934 • Fax: 011-49344935
E-mail: publishing@cbspd.com • publicity@cbspd.com

Branches:

- ***Bengaluru:*** 2975, 17th Cross, K.R. Road, Bansankari 2nd Stage, Bengaluru - 70 • Ph: +91-80-26771678/79 • Fax: +91-80-26771680 E-mail: cbsbng@gmail.com, bangalore@cbspd.com
- ***Chennai:*** No. 7, Subbaraya Street, Shenoy Nagar, Chennai - 600030 Ph: +91-44-26681266, 26680620 • Fax: +91-44-42032115 E-mail: chennai@cbspd.com
- ***Kochi:*** Ashana House, 39/1904, A.M. Thomas Road, Valanjambalam, Ernakulum, Kochi • Ph: +91-484-4059061-65 Fax: +91-484-4059065 • E-mail: cochin@cbspd.com
- ***Kolkata:*** 6-B, Ground Floor, Rameshwar Shaw Road, Kolkata - 700014 Ph: +91-33-22891126/7/8 • E-mail: kolkata@cbspd.com
- ***Mumbai:*** 83-C, Dr. E. Moses Road, Worli, Mumbai - 400018 Ph: +91-9833017933, 022-24902340/41 • E-mail: mumbai@cbspd.com

Representatives:

• Bhubaneswar	0-9911037372	• Hyderabad	0-9885175004	• Jharkhand	0-9811541605
• Nagpur	0-9021734563	• Patna	0-9334159340	• Pune	0-9623451994
• Uttarakhand	0-9716462459	• Dhaka (Bangladesh)	01912-003485		

Printed at:
J.S. Offset Printers, Delhi (India)

● Study Skills

● Why effective study is essential to students of pharmacy?

A student of pharmacy has to study many subjects and techniques during his/her course of DPharm, BPharma, or MPharm, with a prime motto of learning. The principles of effective study help in effective and result-oriented learning to understand the concept of disease, treatment methods and medicines. Wrong information can lead to serious problems to patients because they trust the pharmacist as a friend, philosopher and guide.

● Why pharmacy student must go for "effective learning"?

Effective learning means **learning** with full of concentration towards a particular subject/topic/concept/theme. It requires the use of intelligence on the part of the learner, definiteness of a purpose or goal and firm-mindedness.

● What is study?

Study means Attention, Retention and Recall a particular topic.

● What is the study rule?

For effective study, one has to prepare well the particular topic/concept, thoroughly understand with mind and body, rehearse the subject many times to recall the information whenever needed in future. The student should have sound mind in a sound body to achieve his aim.

● How to make one's learning effective?

Every pharmacy student has to practise the good study habits by getting up early in the morning and studying with a planned time-table to master the subject-matter with good attitude and interest.

● How to cultivate the good learning habit?

Love to study with pleasure not with pressure developing self-discipline, interest in a particular field, read the material rapidly and accurately, observe, listen and gain experience directly, communicate ideas in speaking and writing, infer, draw conclusions, and apply them to new situations. More than anything worthwhile is using free time productively.

● What are the principles and techniques of effective study?

Learning with the heart is a self-active process. Students have to study by their physical and psychological pressures towards that topic/subject by their own efforts and self-realisation. By way of adopting and goal-oriented intelligent learning, one who has a clear vision learns better than the one who does not have.

● What are the techniques of effective study?

1. Purpose of study and problem-solving mind.
2. Organising the daily routine from 5 AM to 10 PM and preparing a timetable for the preparation of the examination.
3. Start the work promptly and with confidence.
4. Every student has to do his/her own preparation for effective study.
5. Collect the study material by survey.
6. Search for essentials in work to look for general principles rather than isolated fact.
7. Make it a habit of discovering interrelationship or connection between one matter to another subject.
8. Prepare small tips/notes.
9. Make small summaries/book cards of important points.
10. Read, review, reread, recite.
11. Give more attention towards important key points, words, definitions, concepts, charts, figures, equations, formulae, chemical reactions, tables, etc.
12. Make small questions and answers to remember; prepare objective type questions and key.
13. Create your own good environment for effective study with a board "Good Luck to Your Studies".

● Crow/Crow and Skinner have enlisted 25 good, result-oriented suggestions for the pharmacy student, who is intended to have good habit of effective study.

1. Study with a definite purpose in hand.
2. Evaluate immediate and remote goals.
3. Provide a definite place for study.

4. See that physical conditions are conductive in study.
5. Plan and follow a definite place for study.
6. Look for the main ideas of reading material.
7. Cultivate the habit of reading rapidly and carefully.
8. Outline the study material.
9. Take brief, well-organised notes in your own language.
10. Evaluate the difficulty of the material.
11. While reading, raise significant questions on the material to be learned, then answer them.
12. Study with intent to recall.
13. Attend carefully to all illustrative material.
14. Complete all study assignments.
15. Let active study and rest period be interspersed with each other.
16. Try to learn the unit or the lesson 'as a whole' when possible.
17. Concentrate on what you are studying at the time.
18. Shut out all emotional distractions.
19. Overlearn sufficiently so that delayed recall is possible.
20. Learn to summarise and review what you have learnt or read.
21. Be alert to ideas emphasised by the teacher.
22. Think over the statements made by the authors and try to challenge them.
23. Find out what the several authorities say about a topic or an idea.
24. Apply the subject matter learnt in as many practical situations as possible.
25. Make intelligent use of the dictionary.

• What is the importance of books?

1. Those who have the books are more successful than the people who do not have books, or are illiterate.
2. Those who have mugged up the knowledge from the books are more successful than the people who have only books.
3. Those who can understand the subject, learn the meaning from the books, and develop the concepts are more successful than the ones who mugg up the topics.
4. The most successful people are those who apply that knowledge in his own field and practise it towards getting perfection.
5. The happiest person is that who loves the job with heart.

What is the importance of talent?

Talent is what a man possesses and the genius is what possesses man. So, to reach the aim, act now only.

Small things:

Small things make perfection, but perfection is not a small thing.

Golden tips for effective reading

1. Dream to earn Rs 2 lakh per month by 2010.
2. Great minds think alike to achieve excellence.
3. Love your studies as you love your parents.
4. Hard work of first 25 years of life fetches next 75 years of happiness and satisfaction.
5. Develop intelligent mind by strictly following daily timetable from 4 AM to 10 PM.
6. Make a habit of reading everyday at the same time, the subject, in same place.
7. No diversion of mind, do *pranayama* for effective learning.
8. Make it a good practice of study with good light and melodious music like *vedaghosha*, *mantras*, prayers, *om mantras*, *Gayathri mantra,* etc. (if you have that habit only).
9. But no music is better. No pop music, it distracts your mind.
10. Have a poster of a person who is reading; it inspires you to study (better a portrait of Swamy Vivekanand).
11. Same place study for good mental preparation.
12. Read by turning towards east or north while light should come from back to fall on your book. Better use table lamp.
13. It is better to discuss with your friends after study and not to mugg up the topics.
14. Do not quarrel with your friends or family members before the study or during the study as it spoils your concentration.
15. If a person disturbs you, kindles you means, smile at him.
16. Make underline the important point.
17. No study after 11 PM.
18. Avoid the **P**ostponement, **L**aziness, **A**bsent-**M**indedness, **TV**, **E**xpressing complaints (**PLATE** disease).
19. Pray to God to help you but remember there can be no dependence

on the *prayer* as there is neither any alternate method to hard work nor any short cut to success.

20. Nonstop reading is not good. Give a 10–15 minutes gap in between study and recall.
21. *Read-Board:* Mind will be stimulated by looking at the board.
22. Take good quantity of water, about 1-2 litres to have a good health.
23. 15 minutes once, change the posture of study.
24. Do not believe that any subject is difficult, rather love the subject so your problem is solved.
25. Do not keep newspapers, magazines, or wall clock in front of you while reading.
26. Cultivate the habit of 'cool' reading and having no tension about examination or no fear of the teacher.
27. Think only on the subject while reading and do not be in a dilemma.
28. For effective learning sit on the floor in *Padmasana*.
29. Definitely have self inspiration like Ekalavya.
30. Dedicate yourself to your work, positive result will come with good appreciation, rewards.
31. Finally you achieve excellence in the chosen field and makes you and your family happy.
32. Real achievement is recognised only when your sound knowledge proves useful to the society and the world.
33. A talented person is like a magnet. He need not go in search of job or money, it will come to him just like that.
34. Your success must give satisfaction and happiness to you and your family and other people should consider you as a successful person.
35. Good skills, knowledge and attitude are the real secrets of your success.
36. Help all, serve all and enjoy everyday life.

Wishing you good luck

Prof. R. Raveendra

R.R. College of Pharmacy
near Chikkabanavara Railway Station
Bangalore 560090

Preface

Welcome to this unique book as a handy companion for all the students of diploma and degree courses in pharmacy. "All men make mistakes, only wise learn from them" is the quote that gains all the more importance as very student makes one or more mistakes in his/her examinations. The only ideal and practical solution for them is to follow a good time table, keep a constant study time in a pleasant study atmosphere. Acronyms in progressing, point-wise and para-wise study, regular self-test, and writing smart answers in examination are the basic steps which get you complete success and bring happiness to you, your family and the society.

Most of the pharmacy students are awaiting a good question bank as there are not many books to solve their problems. I have written this book to meet their demands and expectations based on my long experience in the field of pharmacy education. I do hope that this book will serve as an excellent study guide for the students to score maximum marks in the examinations and to remember the subjects for the future reference in the field of pharmacy.

Prof. R. Raveendra
R.R. College of Pharmacy
Bangalore 560090

Contents

- *Study Skills* v
- *Preface* x

Section A
VIVA VOCE QUESTIONS
Including Practical-Oriented Questions

1. Pharmaceutics I	2–10
2. Pharmaceutical Chemistry I	11–19
3. Pharmacognosy	20–27
4. Biochemistry and Clinical Pathology	28–35
5. Human Antomy and Physiology	36–47
6. Health Education and Community Pharmacy	48–74

Section B
MODEL QUESTIONS
Based on Board Examination Papers

7. Pharmaceutics I	76–77
8. Pharmaceutical Chemistry I	78–80
9. Pharmacognosy	81–82
10. Biochemistry and Clinical Pathology	83–84
11. Human Anatomy and Physiology	85–87
12. Health Education and Community Pharmacy	88–90

Section C
QUESTION BANK
Selected Questions of Paper-Setters' Choice

13. Question Bank	92–138

Acknowledgments

My sincere thanks to all the professionals who assisted me in the development of this reference; the reviewers who gave their perspectives of the comments, insightful suggestions and contributions; and the management, teaching and nonteaching staff of Raman College of Pharmacy, Bangalore, for their moral support.

Thanks are also due to Dr LVG Naragundh, Dr MD Karvekar, Prof TV Narayana, Mr C Basavaraja, Mr R Ajareddy, Dr B Gopalkrishna, Prof BG Shivananda, Prof Chinnaswamy, Mr DA Gundurao and many office-bearers of APTI, IPA, IPGA, KSPC, Saraswathi online.com, etc. My appreciation and love to my family members for their ongoing support.

I am dedicating this book to **Dr. B Suresh,** the youngest and the most dynamic President of the Pharmacy Council of India, and to all the current and future pharmacy professionals of India.

Prof. R. Raveendra

Section A

VIVA VOCE QUESTIONS
(Including Practical-Oriented Questions)

1

PHARMACEUTICS I

I. TABLET

1. Define a tablet.
2. Name the different categories of excipients used in the preparation of compressed tablets.
3. What does the term Slug mean?
4. Name the various diluents commonly used in the formulation of a tablet.
5. Why are binding agents required in certain types of tablets?
6. What are the advantages and disadvantages of tablets?
7. Name various quality control tests for the tablet.
8. Name various stages in sugar coating of tablet.
9. Give advantages of film coating of tablet.
10. Classify different types of tablets.
11. Mention the common defects, which can occur in compressed tablet.
12. What is microencapsulation process?
13. Why is the powdered medicament not compressed as such in tablet form?
14. What are compressed tablets?
15. Why coating is required for the tablets?

II. CAPSULES

16. Define capsule.
17. Name the different ingredients used in the preparation of hard gelatin capsules.

18. What are the various ingredients used in the preparation of soft gelatin capsules?
19. What are the advantages of capsules?
20. Explain packaging and storage of capsules.
21. Give difference between hard gelatin and soft gelatin capsules.
22. Mention quality control test for capsule.

III. DOSAGE FORM

23. Define the term drug.
24. Explain the term unit dosage form.
25. Why liniments should not be applied to broken skin?
26. Give three examples of monophasic liquid dosage form.
27. Why glycerine is used as a base in throat paint?
28. What are the additives needed in preparing different dosage form?
29. What are syrups?
30. What is the difference between elixir and syrup?
31. What are pills?
32. Define container.
33. Define closure.
34. Why closures are necessary to close the container?
35. What are the qualities of good container?
36. Name two examples for biphasic liquid dosage form.
37. Name two semi solid dosage form.
38. How will you distinguish w/o and o/w emulsion?
39. What should be the qualities of ideal suspension?
40. What do you mean by dusting powders?
41. What are mouth washes?
42. Give the advantages of liquid dosage form.
43. What is inhalation?
44. What do you mean by pharmacopoeia.
45. Give difference between lotion and liniments.
46. What are aerosols?
47. Name various parts of aerosol container.

IV. PACKING

48. Mention the basic qualities of neutral glass.
49. Name different types of material used for making of containers.
50. Give the advantages and disadvantages of plastic.
51. Define container.
52. Define closure.
53. Why closures are necessary to close the container?
54. What are the qualities of good container?
55. What is the composition of glass?
56. What is lime soda glass?
57. Name various closures used in pharmacy.

V. SIZE REDUCTION AND SIZE SEPARATION

58. Define the term comminution.
59. What does the term levigation means?
60. Define the term elutriation.
61. Name different modes of size reduction.
62. Name the mill in which size reduction is done by compression.
63. Name the mills in which size reduction is done by attrition.
64. Name the mills in which size reduction is done by impact.
65. What are advantages of ball mill?
66. Give importance of particle size in pharmacy.
67. Mention the various grades of powder.
68. Define the term size separation.
69. What is the importance of size separation in pharmacy?
70. Name various types of separators.
71. Give the principle behind the ball mill.

VI. MIXING AND HOMOGENIZATION

72. Define the term mixing.
73. What are the different equipments used for mixing of powders?
74. Name different equipments used for mixing of liquids.
75. What is the objective of mixing?
76. What does the term viscosity means?

VII. EXTRACTION

77. What are the various processes used in the extraction of crude drugs?
78. What does the term extraction means?
79. Define the term menstrum.
80. What are the advantages and disadvantages of water as a solvent?
81. Name different types of maceration process.
82. What is the difference between maceration process and infusion process?
83. What is double maceration?
84. What is multiple maceration?
85. Name certain ayurvedic dosage form.
86. What do you mean by Bahamas?

VIII. HEAT PROCESS, EVAPORATION AND DISTILLATION

87. Define the term heat.
88. What do you mean by sublimation?
89. What is evaporation?
90. Differentiate between natural circulation evaporators and forced circulation evaporators.
91. What are the various factors, which effect evaporation of a liquid?
92. Define the term distillation.
93. Name the different types of distillation?
94. What is purified water?
95. Define the term water for Injection.
96. Name the dissolved gases present in water.
97. How will you separate two miscible liquids?
98. Differentiate between evaporation and distillation.
99. Define the term drying.

IX. DRYING AND STERILIZATION

100. Name various types of dryers.
101. Differentiate between sterilization and disinfections.

102. Classify the different method of sterilization.
103. Write the advantages and disadvantages of dry heat sterilization.
104. What do you mean by tantalization?
105. What do you mean by pasteurization?
106. What do you mean by aseptic techniques?
107. Define Antiseptics and bactericide.
108. Differentiate between bactericide and bacteriostastic?
109. How will you sterilize the fixed oils?

X. IMMUNITY

110. Define the term immunity.
111. Differentiate active immunity and passive immunity.
112. What are vaccines?
113. What is natural immunity?
114. What do you mean by immunization.

XI. PRACTICAL ORIENTED QUESTIONS

115. Define aromatic waters.
116. Give one example of rubifacient.
117. Define solution.
118. Mention the differences between liniment and lotion.
119. Give one example of lubricant purgative.
120. Mention the names of various flavouring agents.
121. What is deodorant?
122. What is demulcent?
123. Mention the dose of peppermint water IP.
124. One part of camphor and soluble in .... parts of water.
125. Absolute alcohol is
    (a) 100 %v/v (b) 95 %v/v
    (c) 50 %v/v (d) None of the above.
126. What is auxiliary label?
127. What is the use of aqueous iodine solution?
128. Weak iodine solution is for internal use. (True/False)

129. Define saponification.
130. Strong ammonium acetate solution I.P should be stored in amber coloured bottle. (True/False)
131. Define spirits.
132. What is the meaning of word QS.
133. Liquid paraffin is fixed oil. (True/False)
134. Cold cream is w/o emulsion. (True/False)
135. What is the meaning of vanish.
136. Mention one market product of vanishing cream.
137. Beeswax is obtained from ....
138. Potassium hydroxide is an example of salt. (True/False)
139. Give one example of humectant.
140. Methyl paraben in an example of colouring agent. (True/False)
141. Talcum powder is generally contaminated with ....
142. Give some marketed products of face powder.
143. What is the principle involved in shampoo?
144. Bentonite is an example for flavouring agent. (True/False)
145. Borax is
    (a) Salt (b) Acid (c) Base (d) None of these
146. Cold cream can be used as
    (a) Emollient (b) Purgative
    (c) Astringent (d) None of the above.
147. What is the difference between fat and oil?
148. What is the advantage of enteric coating?
149. Potassium iodide decreases the solubility of iodine in water. (True/False)
150. $KMnO_4$ is the formula of
    (a) Potassium permanganate (b) Potassium dichromate
    (c) Potassium per chlorate (d) None of the above
151. What is the difference between disinfectant and antiseptic?
152. A drug that suppresses cough is called
    (a) Anesthetic (b) Antihistamine
    (c) Anti tussive (d) Analgesic

153. Caster oil contains
   (a) Resonolic acid (b) Acetic acid
   (c) Ascorbic acid (d) Salicylic acid
154. Simple syrup is .... solution of .... in water.
155. The emulsion meant for external use should be .... type.
156. The first edition of the pharmacopoeia of India was published in .... year.
157. The first USP was published in .... language.
158. One kilogram is equal to
   (a) 2.2 Pound (b) 2.4 Pound (c) 2.6 Pound (d) 2.0 Pound.
159. Define isotonic, hypertonic and hypotonic solution.
160. Airtight containers are also called .... containers.
161. Containers meant for storage of injectables are made of .... glass.
162. The deficiency of a ball mill is maximum at
   (a) Low speed (b) High speed
   (d) 2/3 of speed (d) Very high speed
163. When the powder is said to be very fine powder.
164. In colloidal mill the motor rotates at a speed of .... to .... pm.
165. Define filtration.
166. What are the advantages of filters?
167. The rate of filtration is .... proportional to the viscosity of the liquid.
168. Describe the terms of: (a) Avalchos (b) Gutikas.
169. Define desiccation.
170. What is the difference between distillation and evaporation?
171. The liquid boils when its .... is equal to the atmospheric pressure.
172. What is the difference between simple distillation and fractional distillation?

173. Liquids which decompose at or below their boiling point are purified by ....
174. What are the uses of spray driers?
175. Proper drying prevents the .... of the product.
176. Define pH.
177. In moist heat sterilization bacteria are killed by ....
178. A substance which can kill bacteria is called
    (a) Bactericidal (b) Bacteriostatic
    (c) Both (a) and (b) (d) None of these.
179. In general the disintegration time of uncoated compressed coated is ....
180. Soft gelatin capsules are made up of ....
181. What is the difference between vaccines and sera?
182. The cholera vaccine contains not less than .... bacteria per millilitre.
183. What is the full form of HIV?
184. An agent that counter acts a poison is called
    (a) Antidote (b) Analgesic
    (c) Purgative (d) Antiseptic.
185. Cachets are usually prepared from a mixture of ....
186. A draught is a liquid preparation taken as a single dose. (True/ False)
187. Emulsions are the monophasic liquid dosage forms. (True/False)
188. Gargles are generally used in .... infections.
189. Give one example of mouthwash.
190. Define suppositories.
191. Mass = ... X volume.
192. One gallon = ... Fluid ounces.
193. One tea spoonful = ... ml.
194. On mixing alcohol with water .... in volume and .... in temperature to get spirit.
195. Ampoules are multi dose containers. (True/False)
196. Define extraction.

197. What is the full form of BCG vaccine?
198. Sterilization by radiation is also known as ....
199. Hot air oven is moist heat sterilizer. (True/False)
200. Define calcinations.
201. Give some examples of filter aids.
202. Convert 1/6 g in to weights.
203. One pint = ... fluid ounces.
204. The international pharmacopoeia is published by the .... organization.
205. Define pharmacopoeia.
206. What is the effect of particle size on absorption?
207. Give one example of lozenges.
208. Give one example of implant.
209. What are pathogens?
210. Give one example of eutectic mixture.
211. Bacteria cause rabies. (True/False)
212. Virus causes cholera. (True/False)

2

PHARMACEUTICAL CHEMISTRY I

I. PHARMACOPOEIA

1. Define monograph.
2. Define pharmacopoeia.
3. Meaning of official compounds.
4. Write the parts of pharmacopoeia in order.
5. Write the years of publication of IP first edition to till date.
6. Name and address of the publisher of Indian pharmacopoeia.

II. ACIDS AND BASES

7. Define buffer.
8. Importance of buffer in pharmacy.
9. Define acids, bases.
10. Name four compounds assayed by neutralization methods.
11. What do you mean by "Physiological acid-base balance"?
12. Mechanism of buffer action with an example.
13. Define Arrhenius theory of acids and bases.
14. Define Lewis theory of acids and bases.
15. Define Lowry-Bronsted theory of acids and bases.

III. ANTIOXIDANTS

16. Define antioxidants.
17. Importance of antioxidants in pharmacy.

IV. GASTROINTESTINAL AGENTS

18. List the official compounds of aluminium and magnesium.

19. Principle involved in the assay of sodium chloride, magnesium sulphate and magnesium trisilicate.
20. Chemical formula and use of bismuth sub-carbonate.
21. Write the preparation of sodium bisulphate and magnesium trisilicate.
22. Use and chemical formula of soda ash.
23. Name official compounds of iron with uses.
24. Define GIT agents with examples.
25. Medicinal uses of calcium carbonate.
26. Define antacids with examples.
27. Define astringents with mechanism of action.
28. What do you mean by antimicrobials with examples?
29. Write on aluminium hydroxide jelly.
30. Medicinal uses of alum and magnesium sulphate.

V. TOPICAL AGENTS

31. Category and chemical formula of alum.
32. Storage conditions and structural formula of borax and boric acid.
33. Medicinal uses of bleaching powder and chemical formula.
34. Principle involved in the assay of hydrogen peroxide.
35. Preparation of ammoniated mercury.
36. Define protective.
37. Preparation of yellow mercuric oxide.
38. Category of sodium potassium tartarate and borax.
39. Storage condition of hydrogen peroxide and potassium citrate, iodine, silver nitrate, chlorinated lime.
40. Role of glycerol in boric acid assay.
41. Importance of 1N sulphuric acid in the assay of hydrogen peroxide.
42. Define with examples equivalent weight.
43. What do you know about "Chelating agent" with an example?
44. Importance of anticaries agent with an example.
45. Importance of tartar emetic.

46. Role of astringent with an example.
47. Role of calamine in beauty care.
48. Importartance of ammoniated mercury.
49. Complete the chemical reaction.
    (a) Lead acetate + Hydrogen sulphide ⟶
    (b) Ammonium chloride + Formaldehyde ⟶
    (c) Silver nitrate + Potassium chromate ⟶
50. Role of acetic acid in the assay of chlorinated lime.
51. Define redox titration with examples.
52. Define iodometry with examples.
53. Explain iodimetry with examples.
54. What do you mean by "Cerriometry"?
55. Give the meaning of "End point" with examples.
56. Importance of "Indicator" with an example.
57. What do you mean by "Equivalence point" with an example?
58. What is the place for "Titrate" in titration?
59. Importance of "White Tile" in titration.
60. What do you mean by "Titration" with an example?
61. "Titrant" where do you fill with an example.
62. Importance of lower meniscus.
63. "Upper meniscus reading to be recorded in colour Titration," why.
64. While titration "Reading to be recorded by holding in hand against to our eye sight level with a good back light"—give reason.
65. Why "To hold the conical flask / iodine flask in right hand and burette cock in left hand"—give reason?
66. Name one inorganic compound as scabicide.
67. Define astringent with example.
68. Define antacid with example.
69. The best available antacid in market.
70. Name some reputed brand names and dosage of emetics, antipyretics, decongesent, astringent.
71. Define with an example protective.

72. What do you mean by "Topical Agents"?
73. Complete and balance by writing chemical equation.
    (a) Cerric sulphate + Ferrous sulphate.
    (b) Hydrogen peroxide + Potassium permanganate + Sulphuric acid.
74. How to test for swelling property of bentonite.
75. Chemical composition and uses of
    (a) Green vitriol (b) Glauber's salt.
    (c) Tartar emetic (d) Talc
76. Name the drug used as fungicide and sedative.
77. Principle in the assay of copper sulphate and magnesium sulphate.
78. Write percentage of weak iodine, Aq. iodine and strong iodine solutions with their uses.
79. Reason of adding potassium iodide while preparing iodine solutions.
80. Give examples and uses of adsorbents.
81. Define with an example expectorant.
82. List saline cathartics, their actions and uses.
83. Balance the equation by writing chemical formula of
    (a) Iodine + Sodium thiosulphate.
    (b) Sodium chloride + Silver nitrate.
84. What do you mean by "Gravimetric analysis"?

VI. DENTAL PRODUCTS

85. Explain the terms—Dentifrices, dental caries, cementum, liners, fillers, mouthwashes and deodorant.
86. Roll of flouries in dental preparations.
87. What is the technique of "Brushing"?

VII. INHALANTS

88. Define inhalants with examples.
89. Storage and labelling of oxygen, nitride and carbon dioxide in cylinders for medical uses.
90. Name the official inhalants with uses.

VIII. RESPIRATORY STIMULANTS

91. What are respiratory stimulants?
92. Importance of ammonium chloride and uses.
93. Role of formaldehyde in assay of NH_4Cl.

IX. EXPECTORANTS AND EMETICS

94. Name the inorganic expectorants.
95. Role of KCNs in copper sulphate assay.

X. ANTIDOTES

96. What do you mean by antidotes with examples?

XI. ELECTROLYTES

97. Category of sodium citrate and importance.
98. Three methods of assay of sodium chloride.
99. Name major intracellular electrolytes.
100. Name major extrtacellular electrolytes.
101. Composition of ORS.
102. Composition of ORS—WHO.
103. Composition of ORS—UNICEF.
104. Define electrolyte combination therapy.
105. Name popular two preparations of combination therapy.
106. How to prepare ORS in home for immediate use with sugar and common salt?

XII. OFFICIAL COMPOUNDS OF CALCIUM, IRON AND IODINE

107. Method of preparation of ferrous gluconate.
108. Synonym of aqueous iodine solution.
109. Storage and use of ferrous sulphate.
110. Preparation of iodine from seaweeds.
111. Official compounds of iron and uses.
112. Official compounds of sodium and uses.
113. Official compound of calcium and uses.
114. Category and formula of calcium gluconate.
115. Official compounds of iodine.

XIII. RADIOPHARMACEUTICALS

116. What do you mean by radioisotopes?
117. Define radionuclides with example.
118. Different kinds of radiations and properties.
119. Different radiopharmaceuticals.
120. What do you know about "Radiopaque contrast medium"?
121. Neat and labelled diagram of GM counter.
122. Define mass number.
123. Biological effects of radioisotopes.
124. Pharmaceutical importance of radiopharmaceuticals.
125. Units of radioisotopes to measure the speed and penetration.
126. Precautions while handling radioisotopes.
127. Who secured Noble prize in radioisotopes?

XIV. QUALITY CONTROL OF DRUGS AND PHARMACEUTICALS

128. Define quality control.
129. Define quality assurance.
130. Differences between "QC" and "QA".
131. Importance of "QA" in pharma industry.

XV. IMPURITIES OF PHARMACEUTICALS

132. Define impurities with examples.
133. Different sources of impurities.
134. How to control impurities?
135. Types of impurities.
136. How the impurities become "Toxic" in pharmaceuticals?
137. In a mixture of good quality rice, basmati rice, salt and stones. Which is desirable and undesirable impurities?

XVI. LIMIT TESTS

138. General procedure for limit test.
139. Define opalescence with example.
140. What do you mean by "Q and Q"?

141. Name the limit test, example for quantative estimation.
142. Name the limit test, compared by "Colour change".
143. Name the limit test, example for qualitative.
144. Name the limit test compared by "Stain".
145. How to prepare "Mercuric chloride paper" in limit test of "Arsenic"?
146. Write on "Gutzeit apparatus".
147. Principle of limit test of sulphate.
148. Importance of aperture in gutzeit apparatus.
149. What do you mean by barium sulphate agent?
150. Principle in lead limit test.
151. Difference between assay and limit test.
152. Principle of limit test of iron.
153. Principle of limit test of lead.
154. Define error.
155. Different kinds of errors.
156. Different sources of errors.
157. Role of nitric acid in limit test of chloride.
158. Role of hydrochloric acid in limit test of sulphates.
159. Principle involved in the limit test of arsenic.
160. Chemical reactions of limit test of arsenic.
161. Give the examples for limit test involving
    (a) Colour comparison
    (b) Stain comparison
    (c) Quantitative LT
162. Role of stannous chloride in stannated HCL IN arsenic limit test.
163. Role of ethyl alcohol and sulphuric acid in barium sulphate reagent.
164. Precautions while doing limit test.
165. What do you mean by "Turbidity"?
166. Stages in limit tests.
167. Why to compare the "Standard solution" with "Test solution" with backside light in LT?
168. Importance of limit test.

XVII. IDENTIFICATION TESTS FOR CATIONS AND ANIONS

169. How to find out the presence of carbonates.
170. Give the identification test for calcium ions.
171. Method of test for sodium ions.
172. How do you test nitrates in any compound?
173. Test for chlorides.

PRACTICAL-ORIENTED QUESTIONS

174. What all the basic requirement for entering pharmaceutical chemistry lab?
175. Precautions to be followed in pharmaceutical chemistry lab.
176. How to handle strong acids and caustics?
177. How to behave in the lab?
178. What all the good laboratory practices (GLP)?
179. What all the precautions before sucking a solution from a bottle?
180. What all the importance of "Measures" and "Labels"?
181. Importance of calibration of glasswares.
182. Importance of weighing in pharmaceutical chemistry lab.
183. Stages of weighing using physical balance.
184. Stages of weighing in analytical balance.
185. Stages of weighing using electronic and sensitive balances.
186. Role of "Rider" while weighing.
187. Good weighing techniques.
188. Good methods of titration.
189. Stages in titrations.
190. What do you mean by acid-base titration, give an example?
191. What do you mean by redox titration, an example?
192. What do you know about complexometry?
193. Importance of first good washing and then only rinsing with same solutions in titration.
194. Items to be carried to pharmaceutical chemistry lab – Must and Should.
195. Why you have to keep "Reagents bottles used" to the same place?
196. Importance of iodometry and iodimetry.

197. Role of droppers.
198. Importance of labelling in pharmaceutical chemistry lab.
199. Importance of use of apron, cap, hand gloves, fuming cupboard, sand bath, oil bath, etc.
200. How to use "Non-luminous" blue flame of bunsen burner?
201. Safety measures to be followed while using gas burners and electrical apparatus.
202. Role of blank solutions and standard solutions in titrations.
203. Importance of periodic table.
204. Conditions to be followed "Strictly" in pharmaceutical chemistry lab.
205. What are the importance of Observation Book, Practical Book and Record?
206. How to mentally prepare for theory and practical exam?
207. Use of "Commonsense" in pharmaceutical chemistry.

3

PHARMACOGNOSY

I. INTRODUCTION

1. Define "Pharmacognosy".
2. Define "Drug".
3. Who is the father of medicine?
4. Name two drugs obtained from minerals.
5. Name two drugs obtained from animals.
6. Name two crude drugs obtained from plants.
7. Define "Hormones".
8. Define "Technical products".
9. Define "Pharmaceutical aid".
10. Name two drugs derived from seeds.
11. Name two drugs derived from leaves.
12. Name two crude drugs derived from barks.
13. Name two crude drugs derived from flowers.
14. Name two crude drugs derived from entire plant.
15. Name two crude drugs derived from exudations.
16. What is staining mixture?
17. Why glycerine is added in the preparation of the slide?
18. Name two alcohol soluble drugs.
19. How will you test for starch in the lab?
20. What is the difference between fruit and seed?
21. What is the difference between root and stem?
22. Define "Distillation".

23. Name the parts of microscope.
24. What is TS and LS?
25. What is difference between organized and unorganized drugs?
26. Define "Standard".
27. What are the types of standards used?

II. CLASSIFICATION OF CRUDE DRUGS

28. Name different system of classification of crude drugs.
29. Name other name for taxonomical classification.
30. Name other name for pharmacological classification.
31. Name two gums containing crude drug.
32. Name mucilage containing drug.
33. Name two crude drugs used as laxatives.
34. Name two crude drugs used as carminative.
35. Name two crude drugs used as GI regulators.
36. Name two pharmaceutical aids and two technical products.
37. Name two drugs of family Leguminosae.
38. Name two drugs of family Umbelliferae.
39. Name two drugs of family Solanaceae.
40. Name two drugs of family Scrophulariaceae.
41. Name two drugs of family Euphorbiaceae.
42. Name two drugs of family Burseraceae.
43. Name two drugs of family Apocynaceae.
44. What is the botanical source of Aloes?
45. Name two animal fibres.
46. Give two examples for umbelloferous fruits.
47. How are drugs classified in IP?
48. What is flavouring agent?
49. Name one animal enzyme.
50. What is the sweetening agent?
51. What are substitutions?
52. Name two crude drugs used as cardiotonics.
53. Name two crude drugs used as astringents.

54. Name two crude drugs used as antihypertensives.
55. Name two crude drugs used as antitussives.
56. Name two crude drugs used as antirheumatics.
57. Name two crude drugs acting an nervous system.
58. Name two antitumour agents.
59. Name one antileprotic agent.
60. Name one antidiabetic.
61. Name one crude drugs used as diuretics.
62. Define astringent.
63. What are diuretics?
64. Define carminative.
65. Name one crude drugs used as antidysentrics.
66. Name two crude drugs used as antiseptics and disinfectants.
67. Name a crude drug used as antimalarial.
68. Name a crude drug used as oxytocics.
69. Name a vitamin containg drug.
70. How are drugs classified in Textbook of Pharmacognosy—Trease and Evans?
71. What is disadvantage of pharmacological classification?

III. ADULTERATION AND EVALUATION

72. Define adulterations.
73. Define evaluations.
74. What is substitution?
75. What is swelling factor.
76. What is extractive value?
77. What is sampling.
78. Define pharmacopoeias.
79. What are the substituents used in senna?
80. What are the substituents used for ispagula?
81. What is importance of ash value?
82. What is swelling factor?
83. Define is ash value?
84. What are substitutions?
85. Give one example for substitution with manufactured material.

86. What are the different methods of drug evaluation?
87. What are the different methods of drug evaluation?
88. What are the different sensory characters observed in drug evaluation?
89. Give one example for substitution with interior material.
90. Name two alcohol insoluble drugs.

IV. CHEMICAL CONSTITUENTS

91. Name one steroidal glycoside-containing drug.
92. Name one saponin glycoside containing drugs.
93. Name two tannins containing drug.
94. Name two volatile oil containing drugs.
95. Name two fixed oil containing drugs.
96. Name two fats containing drugs.
97. Name one wax-containing drug.
98. Name two resins containing drugs.
99. Name two oleoresins.
100. Name two-oleo gum resin.
101. Define alkaloid.
102. Define glycoside.
103. What are carbohydrates?
104. What are resins?
105. What is the difference between volatile oils and fixed oils?
106. What are lipids?
107. Define proteins.
108. Classify carbohydrates.
109. Name four identifying test for alkaloids.
110. Name two identifying test for glycosides.
111. Name two identifying test for resins.
112. Name two identifying test for carbohydrates.
113. Name two identifying test for tannins.
114. Define saponification.
115. What are waxes?

116. Classify tannins.
117. What is salivanoff's test?
118. How are alkaloids isolated?
119. What is nitric acid test?
120. What is the other name for anthraquinone test?
121. Discuss modified Borntragor's test.
122. What is the other name for modified antraquinone test?
123. What is Wagner's reagent?
124. What is borax test?
125. What is combined umbelliferone test.
126. What is Hagger's reagent?
127. What is Mayer's reagent?
128. What is Dregandroff's reagent?
129. Name two examples for isoquinoline alkaloid.
130. Define monosaccarieds?
131. What are monosaccarieds?
132. What are sugars?
133. What are disaccharides?
134. What is cardiac glycoside?
135. What are polysaccharides?
136. What is molish test?
137. What are anthracene glycosides?
138. Name the important chemical constituents of rauwolfia.
139. Give two examples for purine alkaloid.

V. CULTIVATION AND COLLECTION

140. How a high degree of quality of drug is maintained?
141. Why crude drugs should not be stored in wooden boxes?
142. How are drugs stored to prevent from attack by insects?
143. Why are drugs stored in cool and drug place?
144. Why chloral hydrate is added in the preparation of transverse section of the crude drugs?
145. How is ergot stored?
146. Why digitalis should be stored in dark and ambered coloured container?

147. Why cod-liver oil should be stored in airtight container?
148. How is opium stored?
149. What happened if temperature is increased in absorbent cotton?
150. Why packing is done for drugs?
151. What is the botanical source for senna?

VI. SUTURES AND LIGATURES

152. What is the difference between sutures and ligatures?
153. What is the difference between absorbable and non-absorbable sutures?
154. How is catgut sterilized?

VII. FIBERS

155. Name two synthetic fibres.
156. Give chemical test to differentiate wool and cotton.
157. Give chemical test to differentiate silk and wool.
158. Give the chemical test to differentiate silk and cotton.
159. Name two plant fibers.
160. What is the botanical source for cotton?
161. What is the botanical source for jute?

VIII. CHEMICAL TESTS

162. Give two confirmatory tests for benzoin.
163. What is the difference between pale catechu and black catechu?
164. Give two confirmatory tests for asafoetida.
165. Give two confirmatory tests for acacia.
166. Give two confirmatory tests for tragacanth.
167. How will you differentiate acacia and tragacanth by chemical test.
168. Give two specific chemical test for starch and agar.

IX. CRUDE DRUGS

169. What is the botanical source for rhubarb?
170. Give two confirmatory tests for myrrh.
171. Which enzyme is present in castor oil?

172. What is the botanical source for ispaghula?
173. Give one test to differtiate agar and acacia.
174. Give the chemical constituent of senna.
175. What are the chemical constituents present in ginger.
176. Give botanical source for senna.
177. What is the botanical source of digitalis?
178. Name the chemical constituents of fennel.
179. What is the botanical source for arjuna?
180. What are umbelliferous fruits?
181. What is the botanical source for acacia?
182. Name the chemical constituents of cinchona.
183. What is the botanical source for tragacanth?
184. What is the morphological and transverse section difference of cinchona and cinnamon?
185. What is the difference between fruit and seed?
186. What is the botanical source for agar?
187. Name one plant enzyme.
188. What is the botanical source for garlic?
189. Name the chemical constituents of cinnamon.
190. Name the chemical constituent of ipecac.
191. Name the chemical constituents of clove.
192. What is the botanical source for vinca?
193. What is the botanical source for cinchona?
194. What is the botanical source for benzoin?
195. What is the botanical source for myrrh?
196. Give chemical constituents for alma.
197. Name a drug containing strychnine.
198. What is the botanical source for neem?
199. What is the botanical source for Rauwolfia?
200. What is the botanical source for Curcuma and Belladonna?
201. Name two drugs containing Vit. C.
202. What is the botanical source for Aconite?
203. What is the botanical source for shark liver oil and alma?

204. What is the botanical source for peppermint oil?
205. What is the botanical source for *Nux vomica*?
206. Name a drug, which has following constituents
    (a) Menthol (b) Ricinolic acid
207. Name a drug, which has following constituents
    (a) Strychnine (b) Vit. C

4

BIOCHEMISTRY AND CLINICAL PATHOLOGY

I. INTRODUCTION TO BIOCHEMISTRY

1. Define biochemistry?
2. Biochemistry term has introduced by scientist name and year.
3. What are bioimolecules?
4. What are macromolecules?
5. What are micromolecules?
6. What are fields of biochemistry?
7. What is basic unit in tissue?
8. What are cell organelles?
9. Write the nucleus functions?
10. Write the mitochondria function?
11. Write the ribosome's function?
12. Write the endoplasmic reticulam functions.
13. Write the lysosome function.
14. Write the plasma membrane function?
15. Write the Golgi apparatus function?

Match the following

Organelle	Maker
16. Nucleus	Galactosyl transferase
17. Mitochondria	Na^+/k^+ ATPase, 5-nucleotidase
18. Ribosome	Acid phosphates
19. Endoplasmic reticlulam	Glucose-6-phosphatase

20. Lysosomes	RNA
21. Plasma membrane	Glucose dehydrogenase.
22. Golgi apparatus	DNA

II. PROTEINS

23. Define proteins.
24. What is composition of proteins?
25. What are protein functions?
26. What are classifications of simple proteins?
27. What are classification of derived proteins?
28. What is classification of conjugated proteins?
29. Write the mineral structure of amino acids?
30. What are neutral amino acids?
31. What are acidic amino acids?
32. What are basic amino acids?
33. What are sulphur-containing amino acids?
34. What are aromatic amino acids?
35. What are heterocyclic amino acids?
36. What are essential amino acids?
37. All naturally occurring amino acids are leavo rotatory, except ....
38. The charge is 0. Since it carries both positive and negative charges is called ....
39. In isoelectric pH the amino acids exist as ....
40. Biurette reagent contain .... chemicals.
41. Biurete reagent produce .... colour.
42. Ninhydrine test produce .... colour.
43. Xantho protein contains .... chemical.
44. Xantho protein produce .... colour.
45. Millions reagent contain .... chemicals.
46. Millions test to produce .... colour.
47. Sakaguchi reagent contains .... chemicals.
48. Sakaguchi test produce .... colour.
49. Lead acetate test is identified as .... amino acids.

50. Tyrosine is gives to ....
51. Histidine is gives to ....
52. Certain amino acids are necessary to detoxification of toxic substance ....
53. Biological value is calculated by the formula is ....
54. Deficience of proteins are caused .... diseases.
55. Some diseases are caused by the abnormal metabolism of proteins.
56. Define carbohydrates.
57. What are chemical compositions of carbohydrates?

III. CARBOHYDRATES

58. Where functions of carbohydrates?
59. Monosaccharide contains .... molecule of sugar.
60. Disaccharides contain .... molecules of sugar.
61. Oligosaccharides contain .... molecules of sugar.
62. Polysaccharides contain .... molecules of sugar.
63. What are heteropolysacharides?
64. What are homopolysaccharides?
65. What is stereoisomerism?
66. What is optical isomerism?
67. What is asymmetric carbon atom ....?
68. Define mutarotation.
69. Which colour is produced in Fehlings test ....?
70. Which colour is produced in Molish test ....?
71. Which colour is produced in Benedict's test ....?
72. Which colour is produced in Tollen's mirror test .... ?
73. Which colour is produced in Barfoed's test ....?
74. Which colour is produced in Saliwanoff's test .... ?
75. Which colour is produced in iodine test .... ?
76. Molish test is useful for identification of ....
77. Fehlings test, Benedicts test, Tollen's silver mirror test are identified .... sugar.
78. Non-reducing sugar dose not answer any three test ....

79. Reducing sugars (disaccharides) to give ....
80. Reducing sugars (monosaccharides) to give ....
81. Non-reducing sugars ....
82. What are causes of diabetes mellitus?

IV. LIPIDS

83. Define lipids.
84. What are functions of lipids?
85. What are simple lipids?
86. What are compound lipids?
87. What are derived lipids?
88. Define fat.

Define the Following Terms

89. Saponificatiion number.
90. Acid number.
91. Acetyl number.
92. Iodine number.
93. Bees wax is generated by ....
94. Lanolin is secreted by ....
95. Write classification fatty acids.
96. Write essential fatty acid ....
97. Saturated fatty acid should be causal by .... disease.
98. Vegetable fats contain more ....
99. Steroids are compounds which have a common structure called as ....
100. Write the male sex hormones ....
101. Write the female sex hormones ....
102. Write the some examples of steroids ....
103. .... disease is occur abnormal fats are present in the body.

V. VITAMINS

104. Define vitamins.
105. What are fat-soluble vitamins?

106. What are water-soluble vitamins?
107. What is deficiency of vit. A .... ?
108. What is deficiency of vit. D .... ?
109. What are functions of vit. D .... ?
110. What is deficiency of vit. E .... ?
111. What is a function of vit. E .... ?
112. What is deficiency of vit. K .... ?
113. What is function of vit. K .... ?
114. What is deficiency of vit. B_1 .... ?
115. What is functions of vit. B_1 .... ?
116. What is deficiency of vit. B_2 .... ?
117. What is functions of vit. B_2 .... ?
118. What is deficiency of vit. B_6 .... ?
119. What is function of vit. B_6 .... ?
120. What is deficiency of niacin .... ?
121. What is function of niacin .... ?
122. What is deficiency of pantothenic acid .... ?
123. What is function of pantothenic acid .... ?
124. What is structure of vit. B_6 .... ?
125. What is chemical structure of vit. A .... ?
126. What is deficiency of biotin .... ?
127. What is functior. of biotin .... ?
128. What is deficiency of folic acid .... ?
129. What is function of folic acid .... ?
130. What is function of lipoic acid .... ?
131. What is deficiency of vit. B_{12} .... ?
132. What is function of vit. B_{12} .... ?
133. What is deficiency of vit. C .... ?
134. What is function of vit. C .... ?

VI. ENZYMES AND COENZYMES

135. What are coenzymes?
136. Write the group transferring coenzymes ....
137. Write the hydrogen transferring coenzymes ....

VII. MINERALS

139. What are principle elements .... ?
140. What are trace elements .... ?
141. What are essential trace elements .... ?
142. What are possibly essential trace elements .... ?
143. What are non-essential trace elements .... ?
144. What is deficiency of iodine .... ?
145. What is deficiency of fluorine .... ?
146. What is deficiency of sulphur .... ?
147. What is deficiency of magnesium .... ?
148. What is deficiency of iron .... ?
149. What is deficiency of chlorine .... ?
150. What is deficiency of potassium .... ?
151. What is deficiency of phosphorus .... ?
152. What is deficiency of calcium .... ?

Match the Following

Minerals	Functions
153. Sodium	for the synthesis of vit. B_{12}.
154. Potassium	perioxidase and catalase helps in corporation of iron in haemoglobin.
155. Calcium	component of carbonic anhydrase for insulin synthesis and pulse.
156. Phosphorus	synthesis of thyroid hormone.
157. Sulphur	synthesis of haemoglobin, cytochrome synthesis.
158. Iron	compent of biotin, cystin, and methionine.
159. Iodine	synthesis of DNA and RNA.
160. Zinc	bone and teeth formation, blood coagulation.
161. Copper	maintenance of acid-base balance contraction of muscle.
162. Cobalt	maintenance of osmotic pressure.

VIII. PATHOPHYSIOLOGY OF BLOOD AND URINE

163. What are functions of blood?
164. Blood contains ....
165. Plasma occupies in blood ....
166. Cells are occupies in blood ....
167. What are abnormalities of RBC .... ?
168. What are abnormalities of WBC .... ?

Match the Following

Abnormal constituents	Disease
169. Protein	Pyuria
170. Glucose	Hematuria
171. Pentose	Jaundice
172. Ketone bodies	Ketosis
173. Bile salts and pigments	Pentosuria
174. Blood	Glucosuria
175. Pus	Protenuria

176. What are abnormalities of platelets?
177. Classified the lymphocytes.
178. Write functions of lymphocytes.

IX. METABOLISM

179. Define metabolism.
180. What is anabolism?
181. What is catabolism?
182. Other name of glycolysis ....
183. Synthesis of glucose from non-carbohydrates source is called ....
184. Conversion of glucose to glycogen ....
185. Break down of glycogen to forn glucose is called ....
186. How many net ATPS are synthesized in glycosis .... ?
187. Glucose-6-phosphate converted into fructose-6-phosphate .... enzyme.
188. Glucose converted into glucose-6-phosphate .... enzyme.

189. Fructose-6-phosphate to fructose-1,6 diphasphate ....
190. Fructose-1,6 diphasphate to glyceraldehyde-3-phasphate .... enzyme.
191. Glyceraldehyde-3-phasphate converted into 1,3-diphospho glycerate by .... enzyme.
192. 1,3-diphospoglycerate to 3-phosphoglycerate by .... enzyme.
193. 3-phosphoglycerate to 2-phosphoglycerate by .... enzyme.
194. 2-phosphoglycerate to phospho enol pyruvate by .... enzyme.
195. Phosphoenol pyruvate to enol pyruvate .... enzyme.
196. Enol pyruvate into keto pyruvate .... enzyme.
197. Keto pyruvate into lactic acid by .... enzyme.
198. What is Pasteur effect?
199. Pyruvic acid is converted into active acetaldehyde by .... enzyme.
200. Active acetaldehyde is converted into acetyl lipoate by the enzyme ....
201. Acetyl lipoate is converted into acetyl CoA ....
202. Lipoic acid is converted into lipoic acid (Oxidised Form) by the .... enzyme.
203. How many ATPs are produced in citric acid cycle?
204. What is disease significance glucose present in the urea?
205. What is the disease significance bile salts and bile pigments present in the urea?
206. Define enzymes.

5

HUMAN ANATOMY AND PHYSIOLOGY

I. INTRODUTION

1. Define anatomy and physiology.
2. A movement where similar surfaces come nearer to each other is known as ....
3. The movement occurs in shoulder, hip is known as ....
4. Study of nervous system is known as myology. (True/False)

II. CELL

5. Mitochondria is also known as ....
6. Lysosomes are also known as ....
7. Plastids are present in animal cell. (True/False).
8. Centrosomes play an important role during cell division. (True/False)
9. Spermatozoon contain .... pairs of chromosomes.
10. Cytoplasm present in the nucleus. (True/False)

III and IV. TISSUES AND ORGANS

11. Define "Tissue".
12. Endocrine glands secrets enzymes. (True/False)
13. Bone is the hardest connective tissue. (True/False)
14. .... is a tissue which has the power of contraction.
15. Involuntary tissue is under the control of will. (True/False)
16. Which tissue of the following form the covering or lining to the free surfaces of the body?

(a) Muscular tissue (b) Connective tissue
(c) Epithelial tissue (d) Nervous tissue

17. Mention the different parts of neuron.
18. Insulin is an example of enzyme. (True/False)
19. Define "Organ".
20. Genital organs are parts of skeletal system. (True/False)

V. BONES AND SKELETON

21. Give one example of irregular bone.
22. The outer membrane covering the bone is called ....
23. How many number of bones are there in human skeleton?
24. Bones of the skull and trunk form the axial skeleton. (True/False)
25. Which of the following is only movable bone in face
    (a) Maxila (b) Mandible
    (c) Nasal bone (d) None of the above
26. Vomer forms the lower part of the nasal septum. (True/False)
27. Glenoid cavity is the characteristic of which bone
    (a) Scapula (b) Collar bone
    (c) Sternum (d) Innominate bone
28. Trochlear notch is present in
    (a) Ulna (b) Radius
    (c) Humerus (d) None of the above
29. Trachea is the characteristic of humerus. (True/False)
30. Xiphoid bone is a part of
    (a) Clavicle (b) Sternum (c) Mandible (d) Maxilla
31. .... and .... are first and second cervical vertebras.
32. Thoracic vertebra body is heart shaped. (True/False)
33. Lumbar vertebra body is big and kidney shaped. (True/False)
34. Innominate bone is also known as .... bone.
35. Acetabeclum is characteristic of
    (a) Femur (b) Tibia (c) Fibula (d) Hip bone

36. Greater tronchanter and lesser troclauter are charactertics of which bone
    (a) Femur (b) Radius (c) Ulna (d) Humerus
37. Patella is an example of sesamoid bone. (True/False)
38. Lateral malleolus is a part of
    (a) Fibula (b) Tibia (c) Femur (d) Humerus
39. .... number of tarsal bones are present in foot.
40. Trapezium is an example of tarsal bone. (True/False)

VI. JOINTS OF THE SKELETON

41. Define "Arthrology".
42. Sutures of the skull and teeth in their sockets are examples of which joints
    (a) Fibrous joint (b) Cartilaginous joint
    (c) Synovial joint (d) None of the above
43. Sternoclavicular joint is an example of
    (a) Hinge joint (b) Gliding joint
    (c) Ball and socket joint (d) Saddle joint
44. Give one example of ball and socket type joint.
45. .... is caused by the deposition of sodium urate crystals in joints and tendons.
46. Dislocation commonly occurs at .... joint.
47. .... is a disease occurring due to degenerative changes in the cartilages of joint.
48. .... joint disorder is an auto-immune disease initiated by microbial infection.
49. Knee joint is an example of
    (a) Glinding joint (b) Pivot joint
    (c) Saddle joint (d) None of the above
50. Humeroulnar joint formed by trochlear notch of ulna and trochlear surface of humerus. (True/False)

VII. BLOOD

51. .... is a specialized connective tissue which is fluid in nature.

52. Blood is slightly alkaline with a pH of about ....
53. Albumin, globulin and fibrinogen are examples of plasma proteins. (True/False)
54. Mention the names of cellular elements of blood.
55. Rouleaux formation occurs due to the .... shape of RBCs.
56. Polycythemia is a condition where there is a decrease in the number of RBCs or haemoglobin. (True/False)
57. Mention the names of various stages in the development of RBC.
58. .... and .... vitamins as necessary for the development of RBCs.
59. The haemoglobin content of body is about .... grams per 100 ml of blood.
60. .... cells secrete an anticoagulant substance called heparin.
61. Thromboplastin converts prothrombon into thrombin this occurs in the presence of
    - (a) Sodium ions
    - (b) Potassium ions
    - (c) Calcium ions
    - (d) All the above
62. Group A contains A agglutinogen and B agglutinin. (True/False)
63. Mention the names of various types of anemia.
64. Hemophilia is caused due to absence of ....factor.
65. .... is a cancerous condition characterized by an over production of white blood cells.
66. Decrease in the number of white blood cells is known as
    - (a) Leukemia
    - (b) Leucocytosis
    - (c) Leucopoenia
    - (d) None of these

VIII. LYMPHATIC SYSTEM

67. Define "Lymph".
68. The lymph that flows through lymphatic vessels present in villi is called ....
69. Mention the names of various lymphatic tissues.
70. Mention the functions of lymph nodes.

71. .... cells are destroyed in spleen.
72. .... gland takes part in the production of T-lymphocytes.

IX. CARDIOVASCULAR SYSTEM

73. Heart is surrounded by an outer covering called ....
74. The opening between left atrium and left ventricle is guarded by .... valve.
75. Coronary artery supplies which part of the body.
    (a) Heart (b) Kidney (c) Liver (d) Spleen
76. Define "Cardiac cycle" and "Cardiac output".
77. Define "Refractory period" and "Rhythmcity".
78. Define "Pulse" and "Blood pressure".
79. Mention the names of various disorders of heart.
80. What are the complications of hypertension?
81. What are the complications of hypotension?
82. An increase in viscosity of blood increases blood pressure. (True/False)
83. Arteriosclerosis is thickening and inelasticity of arteries. (True/False)
84. Aneurysm is local abnormal dilation of an artery. (True/False)

X. RESPIRATORY SYSTEM

85. Define "Respiration"
86. Mention the names of various parts of respiratory system.
87. .... is a serous membrane which covers the lungs.
88. Inspiration is passive process. (True/False)
89. Expiration is active process. (True/False)
90. Normal value of total lung capacity is ....
91. Exchange of gases between tissues and blood is called as ....
92. Exchange of gases between alveoli and blood is called as ....

XI. URINARY SYSTEM

93. Which is the functional and structural unit of kidney
    (a) Nephron (b) Neuron
    (c) Muscle (d) None of the above

94. Mention the names of various parts of urinary system.
95. .... ml of glomerular filtrate is formed per minute.
96. The capacity of urinary bladder is .... ml.
97. Mention the names of various oedemas.
98. Cessation of urine is called anurea. (True/False)
99. The pH of urine is 11.6. (True/False)

XII. THE MASCULAR SYSTEM

100. Occipitofrontalis is the muscle of the ....
101. Deltoid muscle which is commonly used for .... injections.
102. Thenar eminence is a prominence situated at the base of ....
103. The pelvic floor is formed mainly by ....and ....muscles.
104. Mention the names of muscles of perineum.
105. Define "Myopathy" and "Cramp"

XIII. THE PHYSIOLOGY OF MUSCLE

106. .... is the junction between a nerve ending and the skeletal muscle.
107. Define "Tetanus" and "Fatigue"
108. Adenosine triphosphate (ATP) is broken-down by the .... enzyme.
109. About .... of the lactic acid produced from glycogen is oxidized to CO_2 H_2O.

XIV. CENTRAL NERVOUS SYSTEM

110. Mention the various parts of brain.
111. Gray matter contains
    (a) Nerve fibers (b) Nerve cells
    (c) Ganglia (d) None of the above
112. .... is an important relay station for the incoming fibers of spinal cord and brain stem on their way to cerebral cortex.

113. .... control the fine movements of the body.
114. .... part of the brain is responsible for maintenance of balance and equilibrium.
115. The crossing of nerve fibers in the medulla oblongata is called as ....
116. Pons contain nuclei for
    (a) 1st, 2nd, and 3rd cranial nerves.
    (b) 5th, 6th, 7th and 8th cranial nerves.
    (c) 9th, 10th, 11th and 12th cranial nerves.
    (d) None of the above.
117. Nuclei of 3rd and 4th cranial nerves are present in the midbrain. (True/False)
118. Medulla oblongata contains nuclei for 5th, 6th, 7th and 8th cranial nerves. (True/False)
119. .... ventricle is present in front of cerebellum and behind ponus and medulla oblongata.
120. Mention the various functions of CSF.
121. The brain and spinal cord are protected by three coverings called ....
122. The nerve responsible for hearing is called ....
123. How many pairs of spinal nerves are arising from spinal cord.
    (a) 30 pairs (b) 31 pairs (c) 32 pairs (d) 33 pairs
124. Enteroceptive organs which receive stimuli from ....organs.
125. Reflex action is concerned with involuntary movements. (True/False)
126. In reflex action the response is not quick and immediate. (True/False)

XV. AUTONOMIC NERVOUS SYSTEM

127. Mention the names of various neurotransmitters.
128. In which system acetylcholine is the neurotransmitter in both preganglionic and postganalionic nerve endings.
129. Dilations of the pupil of eye is called ....
130. Constriction of the pupil of eye is called ....
131. Parasympathetic nervous system is responsible for decrease in glandular secretions. (True/False)

132. Alpha receptors, the action on which is excitatory (except intestine). (True/False)

XVI. ORGANS OF SPECIAL SENSES

133. Lacrimal apparatus concerned with the production of ....
134. Choroid lines the posterior compartment of lens and lies between the inner surface of .... and ....
135. The surpensory ligament of lens is attached to .... muscle.
136. 'Rods and cones' are present on the outer surface of ....
137. .... is the fluid present in the both the anterior and posterior chambers of eye.
138. ....and .... regulate the amount of light entering the eye.
139. Unless properly treated glaucoma may lead to .... due to retinal damage.
140. Opacity of the lense is called ....
141. Tympanic membrane is present in
     (a) External ear (b) Middle ear
     (c) Internal ear (d) None of the above
142. Sound waves in air are collected by .... part of the ear.
143. The auditory ossecles which are three small bones arranged across the
     (a) External ear (b) Middle ear
     (c) Internal ear (d) None of the above
144. Each semicircular canal has an enlarged end called ....
145. Match the following

1. Sweet taste	a. Tip of the tongue
2. Bitter taste	b. Front edge of the tongue
3. Sour taste	c. Back of the tongue
4. Salt taste	d. Back edge of the tongue

146. The sensory nerves of smell are .... nerves.

XVII. SKIN AND REGULATION OF BODY TEMPERATURE

147. .... and .... are maintain the texture of the skin.

148. .... muscles are responsible for the straightening of the hair.
149. Define sensible and insensible perspiration.
150. The normal body temperature .... °C.
151. Pain arising from liver is felt in the skin of right shoulder. It is called as
    (a) Cuteneous pain (b) Headache
    (c) Referred pain (d) None of the above
152. Evaporation of sweat makes the skin cool and leads to
    (a) Heat loss (b) Heat gain
    (c) No change in heat (d) None of the above

XVIII. DIGESTIVE SYSTEM

153. Mention the names of various parts of digestive system.
154. Which is the hardest part of the tooth?
155. Which enzyme is present in saliva?
156. Mention the names of different parts of pharynx.
157. .... is the enzyme which curdles the milk.
158. Which is having antiseptic action in gastric juice?
    (a) HCL (b) Pepsin (c) Gastrin (d) Rennin
159. .... is the content of gastric juice which is necessary for the absorbance of vit. B_{12}.
160. Which is responsible for conversion of trypsinogen to trypsin?
    (a) Enterokinase (b) Erepsin
    (c) Maltase (d) None of the above
161. .... organ is the waste organ in GIT.
162. Define "Defecation".
163. The folds of peritoneum connected to the stomach are called ....
164. .... and .... parts of peritoneum serve as storehouse for fat.

XIX. ACCESSORY ORGANS OF DIGESTION

165. .... is the largest abdominal organ.
166. .... is a pear shaped storage sac for bile.

167. .... ml of bile is secreted by liver per day.

168. Capacity of the gall bladder

(a) 30 ml (b) 100 ml (c) 200 ml (d) None of the above

169. What is the anatomical position of pancreas?

170. What is the composition of pancreatic juice?

171. Mention the names of hormones secreted by pancreas.

XX. METABOLISM, DIET AND VITAMINS

172. Define the terms anabolism, catabolism and metabolism.

173. Define calorie.

174. Define basal metabolism.

175. .... liters of water is taken every day.

176. The total body content of iron is about .... gms.

177. In normal diet the ratio of protein, fat and carbohydrate is

(a) 1:1:3 (b) 1:1:2 (c) 2:1:3 (d) 3:2:1

178. Bacteria present in the intestine synthesize

(a) Vit. K (b) Vit. C (c) Vit. D (d) Vit. A

179. .... and ....vitamins deficiency leads to megaloblastic anemia.

180. Beriberi is caused by the deficiency of which vitamin

(a) Vit. B_1 (b) Vit. B_2 (c) Vit. B_{12} (d) Vit. C

XXI. ENDOCRINE SYSTEM

181. Endocrine glands secrete

(a) Hormones (b) Enzymes

(c) Lymph (d) None of the above

182. Which is the master endocrine gland?

183. Vasopressin is the hormone secreted by

(a) Anterior pituitary (b) Posterior pituitary

(c) Adrenal gland (d) Thyroid gland

184. Hypopituitarism leads to

(a) Dwarfism (b) Gigantism

(c) Goiter (d) None of the above

185. The secretion of thyroid hormones is controlled by .... hormones of anterior pituitary.
186. What are the symptoms of Graves's disease?
187. A decrease in calcium level of plasma increases the secretion of .... hormone and vice versa.
188. Which hormone is responsible for fight or flight.
189. Glucogan and insulin having same pharmacological actions. (True/False)
190. .... is a very small gland situated in the brain.
191. Cortisol, cortisone and carticosterone together called
    (a) Glucocorticoids (b) Mineralocorticoids
    (c) Neurotransmitters (d) None of the above
192. Hypo function of adrenal cortex produces .... disease.
193. Aldosterone and desoxycorticosterone are known as
    (a) Glucocorticoids (b) Mineralocorticoids
    (c) Enzymes (d) None of the above
194. Mention the gland name, which is having both exocrine and endocrine nature.

XXII. REPRODUCTIVE SYSTEM

195. .... are the male reproductive organs, which produce spermatozoa.
196. Semen acts as a vehicle for spermatozoa and also it provides .... to the spermatozoa.
197. Each ml of semen normally contains about .... millions of spermatozoa.
198. Milk secretion is stimulated by .... hormone of anterior pituitary.
199. .... hormone of posterior pituitary is responsible for milk ejection.
200. .... is a thin membrane, which covers the vaginal orifice of virgin women?
201. Mention the names of different internal genital organs.

202. Puberty usually occurs in girls at the age of
    (a) 10–14 years (b) 20–25 years
    (c) 5–10 years (d) None of the above
203. After discharging ovum, the graffian follicle form ....
204. Mention the various phases of menstrual cycle.
205. Menopause occurs in women generally at the age of
    (a) At about 45 years (b) At about 60 years
    (c) At about 35 years (d) None of the above
206. Define "Fertilization".
207. The total number of chromosomes in man are ....
208. Placenta is formed by about .... week of pregnancy.

6

HEALTH EDUCATION AND COMMUNITY PHARMACY

I. IMPORTANT TERMS AND DEFINITIONS

Define the Following Terms

1. Health education.
2. Infectious agent.
3. Carriers.
4. Incubation period.
5. Quarantine.
6. Endotoxin.

Fill in the blanks

7. Community pharmacy is a ....
8. The disease transmitted by articles like towel and pen, etc. is known as ....
9. Harmful substance produced in the body by an infecting microorganism is known as ....
10. .... disease is introduced from a foreign land.
11. Presence of roundworm in the tissue or surface of the body is ....

Multiple Choice Questions

12. Transmission of disease through flies is known as
    (a) Vector born disease (b) Fomite born disease
    (c) All the above (d) None of the above.

Differences

13. What is the difference between endemic, epidemic and pandemic?
14. What is the difference between contagious disease and communicable disease?
15. Difference between endotoxin and exotoxin.
16. Difference between epizootic and zoonotic.

II. CONCEPT OF HEALTH

Define the Following Terms

17. Health.
18. Life expectancy at birth.
19. Disease.
20. Primary prevention.
21. Secondary prevention.
22. Tertiary prevention.
23. Physical health.
24. Mental health.
25. Social health.
26. Spiritual health.
27. Nutrient agents.
28. Physical health.
29. Chemical agents.
30. Mechanical agents.
31. Social agents.
32. Disease agents.

Fill in the blanks

33. Physical health shows that all body organs are .... and .... in a normal state.
34. Mental health relates to the .... of the individual.
35. Health is a .... human right.
36. Sickness refers to a state of .... dysfunction.

37. .... is a period before the onset of disease in man.
38. The first link in the chain of disease transmission is a ....
39. The .... is considered as soil and .... as seed.
40. The nutritional agents include ....
41. Disease occurs as a result of .... between the causative agent, host and the environment.
42. Endogenous agents are produced in the .... and their .... may lead to disease.

Multiple Choice Questions

43. "A state of complete physical, mental and social well-being and not merely the absence of disease or infirmity." This definition of health is given by
    (a) UNESCO (b) UNICEF
    (c) WHO (d) Red Cross.
44. "Physical quality of life index" consolidates following three indicators, except
    (a) Infant mortality rate (b) Life expectancy at one year
    (c) Maternal mortality rate (d) Literacy rate
45. Which of the following is not an indicator of mortality
    (a) Doctor population ratio (b) Infant mortality rate
    (c) Expectation of life (d) Literacy rate
46. The most universally accepted indicator of health status of the whole population is
    (a) Crude death rate (b) Infant mortality rate
    (c) Maternal mortality rate (d) Child mortality rate
47. All of the following are morbidity indicators, except
    (a) Incidence rate (b) Prevalence rate
    (c) Disability rate (d) Duration of stay in hospital
48. Secondary prevention of diseases is
    (a) Specific protection (b) Health promotion
    (c) Early diagnosis and treatment (d) Rehabilitation
49. Epidemiological triad is
    (a) Agent, host, environment
    (b) Agent, vector, host

(c) Vector, carrier, environment
(d) Agent, treatment, environment

50. State of social dysfunction is known as
(a) Disease (b) Sickness
(c) Illness (d) None of the above

51. The phase of pathogenesis in the natural history of disease starts when
(a) agent, host, environment interact
(b) disease agent enters human host
(c) signs and symptoms appear
(d) none of the above

52. Which of the following is tertiary level of prevention
(a) Health promotion (b) Chemoprophylaxis
(c) Rehabilitation (d) Early diagnosis and treatment

53. The web of causation for chronic diseases implies that the disease cannot be controlled unless.
(a) All multiple causes are removed
(b) Chain of causation is controlled
(c) A number of multiple causes are controlled
(d) None of the above

54. Prophylactic administration of vit. A in a child is
(a) Health (b) Specific protection
(c) Treatment (d) Rehabilitation

55. Arrange the following in sequence
I. Disability
II. Handicap
III. Impairment
(a) I, II, III (b) II, I, III
(c) II, III, I (d) III, I, II

Difference

56. What is difference between morbidity and mortality?
57. What is difference between prepathogensis and pathogenesis?

III. NUTRITION AND HEALTH

Define the Following Terms

58. Essential amino acid.
59. Proteins.
60. Minerals.

Fill in the blanks

61. The deficiency of vitamin C produces ....
62. .... vitamins can be stored in the body.
63. .... are protective foods.
64. Proteins constitute about .... of body weight in an adult.
65. Diets high in fat increase the risk of ....
66. .... is the only carbohydrate of animal origin.
67. Vitamin A is also known as ....
68. Vitamin K is found mainly in ....
69. 98% of body calcium is found in ....
70. .... is the main store of copper?
71. The sources rich in iodine are ....
72. .... is required for the formation of dental enamel.
73. .... maintain the osmotic pressure.
74. .... is the indigestible component of carbohydrate.
75. The primary function of iron is to form ....

Multiple Choice Questions

76. The body building foods are all, except
    (a) Fruits (b) Milk (c) Pulses (d) Poultry
77. All are essential amino acids, except
    (a) Leucine (b) Lysine (c) Phenyl amine (d) Tyrosine
78. All are nonessential amino acids, except
    (a) Tyrosine (b) Serine (c) Glycine (d) Valine
79. Primary functions of proteins are all, except
    (a) Body building (b) Repair and maintenance
    (c) Antibody formation (d) Providing energy

80. Cereal proteins are deficient in
    (a) Methionine (b) Lysine (c) Tryptophen (d) Leucine
81. Pulse proteins are deficient in
    (a) Methionine (b) Lysine (c) Threonine (d) Leucine
82. Deficiency of lysine in cereals and methionine in pulses can be improved by combining both is an example of
    (a) Essential amino acids (b) Supplementary action
    (c) Nonessential amino acids (d) Limiting amino acids
83. All the following are saturated fatty acids, except
    (a) Lauric acid (b) Palmitic acid
    (c) Oleic acid (d) Stearic acid
84. Which of the following has the highest amount of polyunsaturated fatty acids
    (a) Safflower oil (b) Soyabean oil
    (c) Ground nut oil (d) Palm oil
85. The most important essential fatty acid is
    (a) Linoleic acid (b) Linolenic acid
    (c) Arachidonic acid (d) Stearic acid
86. All are disaccharides, except
    (a) Sucrose (b) Lactose
    (c) Galactose (d) Maltose
87. Indigestible component of carbohydrate with no nutritive value is
    (a) Starch (b) Cellulose
    (c) Galactose (d) None of above
88. Which of the following is the carbohydrate of animal origin
    (a) Glucose (b) Sucrose (c) Starch (d) Glycogen
89. One gram of carbohydrate provides energy
    (a) 4.75 k Cal (b) 9.3 k Cal (c) 4.1 k Cal (d) 3.75 k Cal
90. All are fat-soluble vitamins, except
    (a) Vit. D (b) Vit. A (c) Vit. C (d) Vit. E
91. Preformed vit. A is
    (a) Retinol (b) Beta carotene
    (c) Alpha carotene (d) Alpha arytenoids

92. How much retinal is equal to one IU of Vit. A
    (a) 0.3 mcg (b) 0.6 mcg (c) 1.2 mcg (d) 2 mcg
93. Earliest sign of vit. A deficiency is
    (a) Conjuctiveal serosis (b) Night blindness
    (c) Bitots spot (d) Keratomalacia
94. Which of the following is a function of vit. D
    (a) Increases absorption of calcium and phosphorus
    (b) Formation of bones and teeth
    (c) Helps in mineralisation of bones
    (d) All of the above
95. Daily requirement of vit. D in pregnancy is
    (a) 2.5 mcg (b) 5 mcg (c) 7.5 mcg (d) 10 mcg
96. Which of the following statement is true about thiamine?
    (a) Essential for utilization of carbohydrates
    (b) In India, rice and wheat are main sources of thiamine
    (c) Lost during milling
    (d) All of the above
97. The most common condition due to Riboflavin deficiency is
    (a) Chielosis (b) Glossitis
    (c) Angular stomatitis (d) Nasolabial dysseborrhoea
98. Foods rich in niacin are all, except
    (a) Liver (b) Meat (c) Groundnut (d) Milk
99. The clinical feature of folic acid deficiency is
    (a) Megaloblastic anemia (b) Glossitis
    (c) Infertility (d) All of the above
100. Which of the following is not true about vit. B_{12}?
    (a) Organometallic compound with cobalt
    (b) Has a role in synthesis of fatty acid in myelin
    (c) Liver is the main storage site
    (d) Absorbed from jejunum
101. Iron content is poor in
    (a) Jaggery (b) Dates (c) Mangoes (d) Milk
102. Major source of fluorine to man is
    (a) Water (b) Cheese (c) Milk (d) Green vegetables

103. Daily requirement of iodine is
(a) 100 mcg (b) 150 mcg (c) 200 mcg (d) 200 mcg

IV. DEMOGRAPHY AND FAMILY PLANNING

Define the Following Terms

104. Demography.
105. General fertility rate.
106. Family planning.
107. Contraception.
108. Density of population.
109. Crude birth rate.
110. Reproduction rate.
111. Proportional mortality indicator.
112. Abortion.

Fill in the blanks

113. There is an .... relationship between fertility and economic status.
114. .... aims to improve the quality of life of the people.
115. A number of .... are associated with advancing mother's age.
116. Depot formulation are ....
117. Lippe's loop is .... shaped device.
118. Abstinence means .... from sexual intercourse.
119. 60–80% of all birth occur within first .... of married life.
120. The contraceptive methods may be broadly grouped into
(i) .... (ii) ....
121. Inert IUDs are usually made of ....
122. Mila-D is available in a package of .... pills.

Multiple Choice Questions

123. Demography includes study of all, except
(a) Fertility (b) Mortality
(c) Social morbidity and marriage (d) Morbidity

124. Family planning is to
   (a) Avoid unwanted pregnancies
   (b) Bring about wanted births
   (c) Regulate interval between two births
   (d) All of the above
125. Age and sex composition of the population can be demon started by
   (a) Bar chart (b) Age pyramid
   (c) Pictogram (d) Histogram
126. High fertility in India is due to
   (a) Universality of marriage (b) Lower age of marriage
   (c) Lower literacy rate (d) All of the above
127. In national demographic goals the NRR is proposed to bring down to
   (a) 1 (b) 2.3 (c) 1.9 (d) 4.2
128. Sex ratio is defined as
   (a) No. of females/1000 males
   (b) No. of males/1000 females
   (c) No. of female births in 1000 in births
   (d) No. of male births per 1000 births
129. Literacy is defined as
   (a) Education up to primary standard
   (b) The person has studied in a school for one year
   (c) The person has passed any two classes from a school
   (d) The person can read and write in one language with understanding.
130. The denominator in crude birth rate is
   (a) Total live births (b) Total birth
   (c) Census population (d) Estimated mid year population
131. Conventional contraceptives are those which
   (a) Are temporary methods
   (b) Require action at the time of intercourse
   (c) Mechanically prevent pregnancy
   (d) Are introduced into the vagina

132. Failure rate of CuT is
    (a) More than 10%
    (b) More than 5%
    (c) Less than 5%
    (d) Less than 1%
133. Third generation IUD's are those which have
    (a) Plastic material
    (b) Copper
    (c) A hormone
    (d) An antispasmodic
134. A combined oral pill is having
    (a) Oestrogen 20 gm and progesterone 0.1 mg
    (b) Oestrogen 30–35 gm and progesterone 0.5 to 1 mg
    (c) Oestrogen 50 gm and progesterone 2 mg
    (d) Oestrogen 100 gm and progesterone 5 mg
135. The contraceptive with least failure rate is
    (a) Condom
    (b) CuT
    (c) Oral pills
    (d) Lippi's loop
136. Combined method of contraceptive is when
    (a) Mechanical and chemical methods are combined
    (b) CuT is combined with mechanical method
    (c) Oral pill is combined with CuT
    (d) Vasectomy and tubectomy are combined

Give the explanation of the following abbreviations

137. DMPA.
138. NET – EN.
139. CBR.
140. GFR.
141. GMFR.
142. ASFR.
143. TFR.
144. GRR.
145. NRR.
146. IUD.
147. IUCD.
148. POP.

149. MTP.
150. CPR.
151. FWP.
152. PHC.
153. BBT.

V. FIRST AID

Define the Following Terms

154. First aid
155. Fracture.
156. Burn.
157. Antidote.
158. Poison.

Fill in the blanks

159. A fracture is a .... break in the normal continuity of bone.
160. In India most of the cases of snakebite poisoning are .... and liquids, etc.
161. Shock may be defined as a state of .... failure.
162. A scald is an injury caused by .... like steam, boiling liquids, etc.
163. .... means damage or death of a part of heart muscle.
164. Wound is a break of continuity of .... or .... membrane.
165. A .... is a covering applied to a wound or to an injured part.

Multiple Choice Questions

166. Choking is the result of the blockade of all, except
   (a) Oesophagus (b) Larynx (c) Pharynx (d) Trachea
167. Neurogenic shock can be caused by all, except
   (a) Spinal injury (b) Spinal anesthesia
   (c) Drugs (d) All of the above

168. In anaphylactic shock th e drug of choice is
    (a) Isoprenaline (b) Dopamine
    (c) Coramine (d) Adrenaline
169. In cobra snakebite the predominant symptoms are
    (a) Oedema, unconsciousness, bleeding
    (b) Drowsiness, weakness, paralysis
    (c) Vomiting, pain abd, oedema
    (d) Myalgia, unconsciousness, vomiting
170. Burns involving 90% body surface area are
    (a) 50% fatal (b) 60% fatal
    (c) 80% fatal (d) 100% fatal
171. EDTA is antidote for
    (a) Arsenic, bismuth (b) Lead, mercury
    (c) Heavy metals (d) Organophosphorus compounds
172. In acute myocardial infarction the most important measure to be taken is
    (a) Strict bed rest (b) Sublingual nitrates
    (c) Morphine or pethidine (d) Oxygen inhalation
    (e) All of the above
173. In cardiopulmonary resuscitation by a single person the ratio of cardiac compression and artificial respiration is
    (a) 15 and 2 (b) 10 and 3 (c) 20 and 2 (d) 25 and 1
174. In fracture all symptoms are present, except
    (a) Unnatural mobility (b) Loss of function
    (c) Skin puncture (d) Pain and swelling
175. Hypovolaemic shock requires
    (a) Immediate fluid replacement
    (b) Immediate intravenous antibodies
    (c) Antihistamines and steroids
    (d) None of the above
176. Muslin cloth is used for
    (a) Cravat bandage (b) Triangular bandage
    (c) Maintaining traction (d) All of the above

177. Magsulph dressing is useful for
   (a) Ulcers (b) Unripe boils
   (c) All injuries (d) None of the above

VI. ENVIRONMENT AND HEALTH

Define the Following Terms

178. Environmental sanitation.
179. Disinfectants.
180. Sewage.
181. Sullage.
182. Chlorine demand.
183. Break point.
184. Residual chlorine.
185. Contact period.
186. Arthropods.
187. Insecticides.
188. Rodents.
189. Rodenticides.
190. Pyrethrum.
191. Zoonotic disease.

Fill in the blanks

192. The components of body and their functions constituted man's ....
193. The diseases are caused due to .... in the delicate balance between man and his....................
194. .... is the prime source of all water.
195. .... wells tap the water from above the first impervious layer.
196. Storage of water beyond .... is not recommended.
197. The disinfecting action of chlorine is due to ....
198. The disinfectant action of chlorine is maximum when the pH of water is ....
199. .... air is necessary for healthy life.

200. .... are biggest source of air pollution in the world.
201. The diseases related to air pollution are .... and ....
202. .... is necessary for efficient vision.
203. The important properties of noise are .... and ....
204. Improper excreta disposal causes ...., and ....
205. The length of septic tank is usually .... the breath.
206. Arthropods are have .... legs.
207. Scabies spreads by .... contact.
208. There are stages in the life history of a mosquito.
209. Majority of houseflies is ....

Multiple Choice Questions

210. Safe water is that which
    (a) Does not harm the consumer after prolonged use.
    (b) Does not have any bad taste or smell.
    (c) Is available in sufficient quantity.
    (d) Is near the houses.
211. Which is not a surface water source
    (a) River (b) Pond
    (c) Stream (d) Spring
212. Ground water has all the following advantages, except
    (a) It is from pathogens
    (b) Requires no treatment
    (c) Available throughout the year
    (d) It is hand
213. All the following are true for a sanitary well, except
    (a) Location is 15–100 metres from the houses
    (b) It has a parapet wall above the ground
    (c) It has a drain for spilled water
    (d) A person can get inside to clean it

214. A good sample of bleaching powder should have
   (a) 10–20% chlorine (b) 25–33% chlorine
   (c) 35–40% chlorine (d) 40–50% chlorine
215. All the following are true for slow sand filter, except
   (a) Occupies large space
   (b) It is washed by scraping
   (c) Bacterial removal is better than rapid sand filter
   (d) Operation is highly skilled
216. Does of alum before rapid sand filtration is
   (a) 1–2 mg/1 (b) 5–10 mg/1
   (c) 4–40 mg/1 (d) 40–50 mg/1
217. The disinfecting action of chlorine is due to
   (a) Chloride atom (b) Chloride ion
   (c) Hypochlorous acid (d) Hypochlorite ion
218. Orthotoluidine test measures
   (a) Chlorine left after disinfect ion
   (b) Chlorine added to the water
   (c) Chlorine needed by water
   (d) Level of pollution of water
219. Horrocks apparatus is used to
   (a) Assess the source of water
   (b) Estimate the chlorine demand of water
   (c) Amount of residual chlorine needed by water
   (d) All of the above
220. Thermal comfort depends upon the
   (a) Amount of air pollution
   (b) Temperature and humidity
   (c) Ventilation
   (d) Amount of automobile pollution.
221. A healthy normal person can tolerate sound up to
   (a) 50–60 dB (b) 60–70 dB
   (c) 70–80 dB (d) 80–90 dB
222. Garbage is refuse from
   (a) The streets (b) The industries
   (c) Kitchen (d) Sewage system

223. The 'water seal' in RCA latrine measures
    (a) 1 cm (b) 2cm
    (c) 3 cm (d) 4 cm
224. Sewage is the waste of
    (a) Toilets (b) All drains and toilets
    (c) Industries and houses (d) Industries and hospitals
225. Sewage farming is suitable for the crop of
    (a) Groundnut (b) Spinach
    (c) Carrots (d) Ladyfinger
226. Insects have
    (a) Two body divisions and three pairs of legs
    (b) Three body divisions and three pairs of legs
    (c) Two body divisions and four pairs of legs
    (d) Two body divisions and five pairs of legs
227. Scabies is caused by
    (a) Ticks (b) Cyclops
    (c) Itch mite (d) Cockroaches
228. Zoonotic diseases are
    (a) Basically animal diseases accidentally transmitted to man
    (b) Diseases of men transmitted to animals
    (c) Diseases transmitted by arthropods
    (d) Diseases transmitted by rodents.
229. Housefly transmits diseases
    (a) Mechanically (b) By participating in lifecycle
    (c) Through its larva (d) Through its eggs
230. Biological control of insects includes
    (a) Growing fungi in water
    (b) Growing fishes in water
    (c) Genetic control
    (d) All of the above

Give the explanation of the following abbreviation

231. DDT.
232. BHC.

VII. FUNDAMENTAL PRINCIPLES OF MICROBIOLOGY

Define the Following Terms

233. Microbiology.
234. Microorganism.
235. Bacteria.
236. Virus.
237. Fungus.
238. Yeas.
239. Moulds.
240. Protozoa.
241. Culture.
242. Colony.
243. Pure culture.
244. Mixed culture.
245. Inoculation.

Fill in the blanks

246. Microorganisms are included in the kingdom named as ....
247. Virus can be seen only with .... microscope.
248. Vibrios are .... shaped.
249. Cytoplasmic membrane of bacterial cell is a closely pack .... layer.
250. Spores are....... in diameter and .... in shape.
251. Algae are a group of .... bearing plants.
252. Fungi have ...... cell wall.
253. The term virus literally means ....
254. Protozoa multiply .... by binary fission or multiple fission.
255. Acid fast staining method was first developed by ....
256. Penicillin was discovered by ....
257. Staining techniques was introduced by ....
258. .... introduced sterilization technique.

Multiple Choice Questions

259. Streptococci can cause all, except
   (a) Rheumatic fever (b) Skin infection
   (c) Meningitis (d) Glomerulonephritis

260. Pneumonia is caused by all, except
    (a) *Pneumococcus* (b) *Mycoplasma pneumoniae*
    (c) *M. tuberculosis* (d) *Bacillus anthracis*
261. All are higher fungi, except
    (a) Ascomycetes (b) Phycomycetes
    (c) Basidiomycetes (d) Fungi imperfecti
262. Commonest media for fungi growth are all, except
    (a) Nutrient agar (b) Sabouraud's glucose agar
    (c) Czapek-Dox medium (d) Cornmeal agar
263. Systematic fungal infections are caused by
    (a) Soil saprophytes (b) Microconidia
    (c) Chlamydiospores (d) Mycelium
264. HIV is a
    (a) DNA virus (b) RNA virus
    (c) Paramyxo virus (d) Retrovirus
265. Bacteria decolorized by acid are
    (a) Gram +ve (b) Gram –ve
    (c) Bacterioids (d) Acid fast
266. Ziehl nelson staining is done specifically for
    (a) Mycobacteria (b) Spirochetes
    (c) Yeast and fungi (d) None of above

Difference

267. What is the difference between gram positive and negative bacteria?

VIII. COMMUNICABLE DISEASES

Define the Following Terms

268. AIDS.
269. Incubation period.
270. Leprosy.
271. Communicable diseases.

Fill in the blanks

272. Influenza is commonly known as ....
273. Poliomyelitis replicates mainly in the .... tract.
274. Cholera comes under .... as well as .... diseases.
275. Spread of *Salmonella typhi* is through .... route.
276. Hookworms are .... belonging to the family ....
277. Plague is primarily a .... disease.
278. Rabies is also known as ....
279. Tetanus is a .... disorder.
280. Chickenpox occurs in children under .... of age.
281. Syphilis is characterized by episodes of active disease interrupted by periods of ....
282. Leprosy is a chronic .... infection of humans.

Multiple Choice Questions

283. Chickenpox is caused by
   (a) Variola virus (b) Varicella zoster
   (c) Rota virus (d) Tanapox
284. Incubation period of measles is
   (a) 5 days (b) 7 days
   (c) 10 days (d) 18 days
285. Influenza spreads by
   (a) Faecal route (b) Droplet infection
   (c) Genetically (d) Mother to foetus
286. Diphtheria antitoxin is given in a does of
   (a) 1000–2000 units (b) 5000–10,000 units
   (c) 10,000–20,000 units (d) 10,000–30,000 units
287. Whooping cough affects children
   (a) 0–1 year (b) 1–2 years
   (c) 2–3 years (d) up to 5 years
288. BCG vaccine in UIP is recommended at the age of
   (a) At birth (b) 6 weeks
   (c) 6 months (d) One year

289. Usual incubation period of amoebiasis is
    (a) 1 week (b) 2–4 weeks
    (c) 1–3 weeks (d) 4 weeks
290. Ascariasis is transmitted by
    (a) Contaminated water
    (b) Contaminated milk
    (c) Raw vegetables and salads
    (d) Flesh food
291. In polio-myelitis cases paralysis occurs in
    (a) < 10% cases (b) < 5% cases
    (c) < 2% cases (d) < 1% cases
292. Hepatitis B is transmitted through
    (a) Parenteral route (b) Sexual route
    (c) Mother to child (d) All of the above
293. For 1 litre of oral rehydration solution amount of common salt needed is
    (a) 1.5 gm (b) 2.5 gm (c) 3.5 gm (d) 4.5 gm
294. Two primary doses of TAB vaccine are given at
    (a) 4 weeks interval (b) 4–6 weeks interval
    (c) 4–8 weeks interval (d) 4–10 weeks interval
295. In food poisoning
    (a) Many persons are affected simultaneously
    (b) Symptoms are same
    (c) History of consuming same food is present
    (d) All of the above
296. Albendazole in ancylostoma infestation is given in a dose of
    (a) 100 mg (b) 200 mg (c) 300 mg (d) 400 mg
297. Source of infection in plague is
    (a) Infected rodents (b) Rat fleas
    (c) Pneumonic plague cases (d) All of the above
298. Radical treatment in malaria is given when
    (a) Fever is present (b) Parasite is present in blood
    (c) Biting mosquito is +ve (d) Fever has lasted for 15 days

299. Filariais causes
 (a) Many deaths (b) Disabilities
 (c) Social stigma (d) None of the above
300. Death rate in rabies cases is
 (a) 50% (b) 70% (c) 90% (d) 100%
301. Incubation period of trachoma is
 (a) 1–2 days (b) 2–5 days
 (c) 5–12 days (d) 10–20 days
302. Human tetanus immunoglobulins are given in a does of
 (a) 150–200 IU (b) 200–500 IU
 (c) 500–1000 IU (d) 1000–2000 IU
303. Leprosy mainly affects
 (a) Nerves and skin (b) Muscles and bones
 (c) Testes and eyes (d) All of the above
304. T. palladium is a
 (a) Very sensitive organism (b) Resists heating
 (c) Bacillus (d) Bacteria of animals also
305. Gonorrhea can be treated easily by
 (a) Penicillin (b) Erythromycin
 (c) Tetracycline (d) Cotrimoxazole
306. HIV virus is
 (a) DNA virus (b) RNA virus
 (c) Tanapox virus (d) Varicella virus
307. HIV is transmitted by all, except
 (a) Sexually (b) Through blood
 (c) From mother to child (d) All of the above

Difference

308. What is the difference between enteric fever and typhoid fever?

Give the explanation of the following abbreviations

309. STD.

IX. NONCOMMUNICABLE DISEASES

Define the Following Terms

310. Noncommunicable diseases.

311. Cancer.
312. Blindness.
313. Hypertension.
314. Diabetes.
315. Coronary heart disease.
316. Stroke.

Fill in the blanks

317. The terms cancer, malignancy and neoplasia are ....
318. Hepatocellular carcenoma due to chronic infection with .... are also known.
319. Diabetes mellitus is a clinical .... characterized by hyperglycemia.
320. Ischemia refers to .... of oxygen due to inadequate perfusion.
321. Blood pressure means .... exerted on the walls of blood vessels by the blood with in them.
322. Rheumatic fever is predominantly disease of .... and adolescence.
323. Blindness is inability to count fingers in daylight at a distance of ....

Multiple Choice Questions

324. The following are the major risk factors for noncommunicable diseases, except
    (a) Smoking (b) Stress
    (c) Alcohol use (c) All of the above
325. Cancers are caused by
    (a) Diatary factors (b) Tobacco consumption
    (c) Exposure to chemicals (d) Viruses and fungi
    (e) All of the above
326. Diabetes mellitus is caused by
    (a) Pancreas diseases (b) Defective insulin formation
    (c) Viral infection (d) Genetic defects
    (e) All of the above

327. Causes of blindness in order of the prevalence are
   (a) Cataract, trachoma, malnutrition
   (b) Malnutrition, trachoma, cataract
   (c) Trachoma, cataract, malnutrition
   (d) Cataract, malnutrition, trachoma
328. What specific factors are associated with Indian population in relation to coronary artery diseases
   (a) Alcoholism and smoking
   (b) Hypertension and high cholesterol
   (c) Genetic and ethnic factor
   (d) Diabetes and oral contraceptives
329. Hypertension is a common cause of
   (a) Coronary artery diseases (b) Stroke
   (c) Blindness (d) All of the above
330. Rheumatic heart disease affects
   (a) Heart and muscles (b) Heart and nerves
   (c) Heart and arteries (c) Heart and joints

X. EPIDEMIOLOGY

Define the Following Terms

331. Epidemiology.
332. Immunity.
333. Immunization.
334. Immunological agents.
335. Nosocomal infections.
336. Cohort study.
337. Reservoir.
338. Susceptible host.
339. Phogocytosis.
340. Vector.
341. Period of infectivity.
342. Incidence.
343. Contact.

344. Exotic.
345. Epizootic.
346. Pandemic.
347. Sporadic.
348. Endemic.
349. Epidemic.
350. Host.
351. Fomites.
352. Contagion.
353. Contamination.
354. Infection.
355. Infectious disease.
356. Mortality.
357. Morbidity.
358. Vaccine.
359. Antigen.
360. Antibody.
361. Toxoids.
362. Antisera.
363. Disinfectant.
364. Antiseptic.
365. Detergent.
366. Deodorant.

Fill in the blanks

367. Epidemiological is the basic science .... of medicine.
368. The health and disease pattern in a community is never ....
369. When an epidemic spread widely is known as ....
370. Immunity is .... the effects of invading pathogenic microorganisms.
371. Natural immunity is due to an individual's .... make up.
372. There are .... major classes of human immunoglobulins.

373. ……………... is the oldest communicable disease control measure.
374. A ……….. is a surface which ……………… the growth of microorganisms.
375. A person with…………. immunity is known as …………... host.
376. Case control study is called as ………………
377. Cohort study is called as ………………

Multiple Choice Questions

378. BCG vaccine is given
   (a) Intramuscularly (b) Subcutaneous
   (b) Intradermally (d) All of the above
379. Autoclaving is a process of
   (a) Heating with chemicals
   (b) Heating under pressure
   (c) Chemical treatment with ionizing radiations
   (d) All of the above
380. UIP includes immunization for all, except
   (a) Tuberculosis (b) DPT
   (c) Influenza (d) Measles
381. Ice lined refrigerators are useful when
   (a) Refrigerator is not available
   (b) Power supply is irregular and limited
   (c) Vaccine carriers are out of order
   (d) Prolonged storage is required
382. A vaccine carrier can keep vaccines safe for
   (a) 12 hours (b) 24 hours (c) 2 days (d) One week
383. Moist heat sensitive vaccine is
   (a) BCG (b) Measles (c) OPV (d) DPT
384. Plasma half-life of IgG antibodies is
   (a) 5–10 days (b) 1–3 days (c) 6–8 days (d) 23 days
385. Polyvalent vaccine is
   (a) Protecting against many diseases
   (b) Having all the types of organisms
   (c) Having toxoid as adjuvant
   (d) None of the above

386. All are killed vaccines, except
(a) Rabies (b) BCG (c) Pertussis (d) Tetanus toxoid

387. Which is not a live attenuated vaccine
(a) BCG (b) Measles (c) OPV (d) Pertussis

388. The process of attenuation is
(a) Separating fractions for vaccine production
(b) Sterilization of the serum
(c) Repeated subculture to remove pathogen city
(d) None of the above

389. Herd immunity depends on
(a) Subclinical infection (b) Immunization status of herd
(c) Herd structure (d) All of the above

390. All are true about active immunity, except
(a) Duration of protection is long
(b) Protective efficacy is more
(c) It is rapidly established
(d) Severe reactions are rare

391. Commonly calculated period is
(a) Incubation period (b) Latent period
(c) Serial interval (d) Generation time

392. Vector is
(a) Arthropod or animal (b) Bacteria or animal
(c) Virus or parasite (d) None of the above

393. Water as vehicle can transmit all, except
(a) Poliomyelitis (b) Diarrhoea
(c) Tetanus (d) Roundworm

394. Vertical transmission means
(a) Transmission from high altitude to low
(b) Transmission from elders to children
(c) Transmission from the rich to poor
(d) Transmission from mother to foetus

395. Reservoir of infection is
(a) Sufferer of the disease
(b) Susceptible to the disease

(c) Chronic case of the disease
(d) None of the above

396. The term 'infestation' refers to
(a) Bacteria (b) Viruses
(c) Rickettsia (d) Arthropods and parasites

397. The following diseases are more common in higher socio-economic classes, except
(a) Obesity (b) Hypertension
(c) Diabetes (c) Anemia

398. Seasonal trend is shown by all, except
(a) Measles (b) Heat stroke
(c) Influenza (d) Accidents

399. Prevalence rate measures occurrence of
(a) New cases only (b) Old cases only
(c) Old and new cases both (d) None of the above

400. Incidence rate is
(a) No. of new cases per 1000 population in an area
(b) No. of old cases per 1000 population in an area
(c) Total number of cases per 1000 population in an area
(d) No. of deaths per 1000 population in an area

401. Epidimiology deals with study of
(a) All health related events and states in population
(b) Epidemic diseases
(c) Communicable diseases
(d) Communicable and noncommunicable diseases

Differences

402. What is difference between infection and infestation?
403. What is difference between toxoid and vaccine?

Give the explanation of the following abbreviations

404. BCG
405. DPT
406. DT
407. TT
408. ATS

Section B

IMPORTANT 200 MARKS QUESTIONS (Model Questions Seclected from Various 10 Years Board Question Paper)

7

PHARMACEUTICS I

1. (a) What is size reduction? Give the importance of size reduction in pharmacy.

   (b) What are the factors, which affects the size reduction of the particles?

2. (a) Discuss various methods of size reduction with the help of the diagram.

   (b) Write a short note on levigation and elutriation.

3. Define size separation, what are the various methods used for size separation of the particles?

4. (a) Define homogenization. Describe commonly used homogenizes. Describe various equipments used for mixing of powders.

   (b) With the help of neat diagram explain various equipments used for mixing of liquids.

5. (a) What is filtration? Explain the theory behind it.

   (b) What are the factors, which affect the rate of filtration, write a note on filter media and filter aids.

6. (a) What are the various filtering devices used in pharmaceutical industry?

   (b) Write a short note on

   (i) Viscosity (ii) Surface tension (iii) Wetting agents

7. (a) What is extraction? Describe the various process of extraction.

   (b) Describe various solvents used in the process of extraction.

8. (a) What are the factors which affects the choice of extraction process?
   (b) Write a note on ayurvedic dosage form.
9. (a) What is evaporation? Describe the various factors, which affects the evaporation.
   (b) Discuss various equipments used in the process of evaporation.
10. (a) Add a note on
    (i) Desiccation (ii) Sublimation
    (b) Define distillation. Describe various types of distillation process.
11. (a) Explain the term sterilization.
    (b) Add a note on test for sterility.
12. (a) Describe the various methods of sterilization.
    (b) What do you understand by aseptic technique?
13. (a) Describe the design of aseptic room.
    (b) Describe various additives used in the preparation of tablets.
14. (a) Define tablet, classify various types of tablet with examples.
    (b) Give advantages and disadvantages of tablets.
15. (a) Describe the process of manufacture of tablets.
    (b) Mention various quality control tests for tablets.
    (c) Add a note on coating.
16. (a) Define capsules, give the difference between hard and soft gelatin capsules.
    (b) What are immunological products, describe advantages and disadvantages of capsules?
17. (a) Define immunity, describe various factors responsible for producing immunity.
    (b) Differentiate active immunity and passive immunity.

8

PHARMACEUTICAL CHEMISTRY I

1. What do you mean by official compounds? Write in detail about monograph IP. With an example from IP 1985.
2. Define acids, bases, buffers with suitable examples, name the compounds assayed by neutralization, physiological acid base balance with example, explain the 6–8 pharmaceutical uses of buffers, chemistry of boric acid.
3. Define anti-oxidants with suitable examples and importance in pharmaceutical industry.
4. List the official compounds with their chemical formula, preparation, structural formula and uses of aluminium, magnesium, sodium, bismuth, iron, calcium and iodide.
5. What are GIT agents? Classify with suitable examples and uses. Define with examples of antacids, astringent and their 2 preparations, uses, chemical structural formula, assay, saline cathartics, adsorbents, fungicide, sedative, antimicrobials, emetic, scabicide, Eq.wt. chelating agent, anticaries agent.
6. Give the formula, uses, storage, preparation and assay of the following iodine, $AgNO_3$, H_2O_2, chlorinated lime, bleaching powder, tartar emetic, calamine, ammoniated mercury, boric acid, alum, borax, lead acetate, magnesium sulphate, green vitriole, Glauber's salt, talc, sodium citrate, $KMnO_4$.
7. Define protective with suitable examples of 2 preparations, assay and medicinal uses.
8. Explain the terms with suitable examples dentifrices, dental products, dental caries, anticaries agent.

9. Define, classify inhalants and explain uses, the preparation, storage, labeling conditions of oxygen, carbon dioxide and nitrous oxide. Add a note on respiratory stimulants and write the preparation, assay and uses of NH_4Cl.
10. Write in detail about expectorants. Explains the role of H-CHO in the assay of NH_4CL, KCNS used in $CuSO_4$ assay, add a note on antidotes and acid-base balance.
11. Write a note on major intra- and extracellular 4- cations and 4- anions, ORS, electrolyte combinations therapy.
12. Give synonym, chemical formula, uses, storage, official compounds iron, ferrous gluconate, iodine, ferrous sulphate, magnesium compounds, sodium and calcium compounds.
13. Define isotopes, radionuclides, mass number of radiopharmaceuticals, properties of alpha, beta and gamma rays, biological effects of radiations, storage and handling of radioactive elements, radioopaque contrast medium and uses of radiopharmaceuticals.
14. Define quality control, quality assurance and their importance in Pharmaceutical industry, sources of impurities, factors to be considered while fixing the limits for impurities in pharmaceutical substances.
15. Define, difference between assay and limit test, describe the principle, procedure, importance of each ingredient in the limit test of chloride, sulphate, iron, lead, arsenic, examples of limit test of chloride, sulphate, iron, lead, arsenic, examples of limit test done to test with colour comparison, stain comparison, quantitative limit test, sources of different kinds of errors.
16. Give the identification tests and chemical reactions of calcium, carbonates, sodium, nitrate, chloride... etc.
17. Give the reasons for the following glycerol in boric acid assay, NH_2SO_4 in assay of H_2O_2, acetic acid in the assay of chlorinated lime, swelling property of bentonite, H-CHO in assay of NH_4Cl, KCNS in $CuSO_4$ Assay, HNO_3 in limit test of chloride, HCl in limit test of sulphate. Role of stannous chloride in stannated HCl in arsenic limit test. Alcohol and H_2SO_4 in barium sulphate reagents.

18. Complete and balance the equation
    (a) Iodine + sodium thiosulphate
    (b) Sodium chloride + silver nitrate
    (c) Ferrous sulphate + cerric sulphate
    (d) Hydrogen peroxide + pot permanganate + sulphuric acid + lead acetate + hydrogen sulphide
    (e) Ammonium chloride + formaldehyde
    (f) Silver nitrate + potassium chromate

9

PHARMACOGNOSY

1. (a) Define pharmacognosy.
   (b) Give various sources of crude drugs with examples.
   (c) Discuss the history of pharmacognosy.
2. (a) Give different system of classification of crude drugs.
   (b) Add a note on various indigenous systems of medicines.
3. (a) Define adulteration. Mention various methods of adulteration.
   (b) Define drug evaluation and discuss various methods of drug evaluation.
4. (a) What are alkaloids? Classify them with suitable examples.
   (b) Give chemical test for alkaloids.
5. (a) What are tannins?
   (b) Define resins and classify different types of resins with examples.
6. Give the pharmacognosy scheme for fennel and coriander.
7. Give botanical source, morphology, microscopy, chemical constituents and uses of *Nux vomica* and ginger.
8. (a) Discuss the collection and cultivation of senna and opium.
   (b) Discuss the life cycle of ergot and also explain its collection.
9. (a) How is digitalis leaves collected for the market?
   (b) How is roulfia collected for market?
   (c) What is the significance of pharmacopoeal standards?
10. (a) What are terpenoids?
    (b) Give the difference between volatile oils and fixed oils with examples.

11. (a) Define fibres. Classify them with examples.
    (b) What are surgical dressings?
    (c) Define sutures how will you prepare suture?
    (d) Give the difference between sutures and ligatures.
12. (a) Draw and explain the morphology and microscopy of Datura and cinnamon and also give its botanical sources, chemical constituents and uses.
    (b) Give the difference between Cinchona and Cinnamon.
13. (a) Give the pharmacognostic scheme of ipecac.
    (b) Give the difference between pharmaceutical aids and technical products.
14. (a) What are enzymes? Describe the various enzymes containing drug with examples.
    (b) Give 2 vitamins containing drug and 2 drugs acting on nervous system. Give the chemical constituents and uses.
15. Give BS chemical constituents for following category of any two drugs.
    (a) Laxative (b) Calamination
    (c) Antiseptic (d) Anti tissue.
16. (a) What are glycosides, classify with examples?
    (b) Add note on cardiac glycosides.
17. Give BS chemical constituents for following categories of any two drugs.
    (a) Antirhumatic (b) Antidiabetic (c) Antidysenteric.
18. Give chemical tests for the following drugs (any two test for each drugs).
    (a) Agar (b) Tragacanth (c) Myrrh
    (d) Acacia (e) Asofoetida (f) Aloes.

10

BIOCHEMISTRY AND CLINICAL PATHOLOGY

1. Discuss biological functions of proteins. Discuss the acid-base behaviour of amino acids. Define proteins. Classify with examples. Write biological value of proteins.
2. What are essential amino acids? Discuss their biological functions. List out names. Write a note on
   (a) Kwashiorkor (b) Marasmus.
3. (a) What are carbohydrates? Classify them with examples. Describe the nutritional functions of carbohydrates.
   (b) What are disaccharides? Write the structure of maltose and give a test to distinguish it from sucrose.
4. Define reducing and non-reducing sugars? Write the structure of glucose and fructose and give one test differentiates them. Explain the following tests.
   (a) Molish test (b) Osazone test.
5. (a) Define the following terms.
   (i) Iodine number (ii) Saponification number
   (iii) Acid number (iv) Acetyl number.
   (b) Define the lipids. Classify them with examples. Write a note on fatty acids? What are there biological functions. Write a note on essential fatty acids.
6. Classify vitamins and name the disease caused by the deficiency of each vitamin. Explain biological functions of vit. D, Vit. K, and vit. C. Write briefly about pellagra and beriberi. What are co-factors and co-enzymes? Write the functions give example.

7. Give sources, chemistry, biological functions and deficiency symptoms of vit. D.
8. Write biological functions of copper, iron, sodium, calcium and phosphorus.
9. Discuss IOB classification of enzymes. Describe briefly special properties of enzymes. Write a note on competitive enzyme in inhibition. Write the mechanism of action of enzyme action.
10. Discuss the effects of substrate and enzyme concentration on the enzyme catalyzed reaction. Write a note on the specify of enzymes. Discuss the effects of pH and temperature on enzyme activity.
11. Discuss reactions at citric acid cycle and its significance and energetic formed. Outline the conversion of pyruvate to acetyl CoA.
12. What is glycolysis? Write with the help of flow chart show the reactions of glycolysis giving energetic under aerobic and anaerobic conditions.
13. Give the account of beta-oxidation of palmitic acid and give its significance and energetic.
14. Explain glycogenolysis, gluconeogenesis. What are ketonuria, ketosis and ketogenesis?
15. Describe the metabolism of phenylalanines and tyrosine gives the importance of HMPS pathway. Write a note on ketone bodies.
16. Explain transamination, deamination, decarboxylation of amino acids with one example for each. What is significance of each trans reaction?
17. Discuss in detail about the abnormal constituents of urine and their significance in disease. What are abnormal constituents of blood and their significance?
18. What are platelets? What is their role of body? What are lymphocytes? Discuss their role in the body. Write principle involved in the test for ketone bodies of the salts.

11

HUMAN ANATOMY AND PHYSIOLOGY

1. (a) Define the following terms.
   (i) Anatomy (ii) Physiology (iii) Histology
   (iv) Health (v) Splanchology
   (b) Define cell and name the different organelles of cell.
   (c) Write short note on mitochondria.
2. (a) Define tissues. Name different types of connective tissues.
   (b) Name the different types of muscle tissue. Discuss the skeletal muscle.
   (c) Name the bones of lower limb.
   (d) Name the bones of the skull.
3. (a) List the functions of bone.
   (b) Explain the identifying features of scapula with a neat-labeled diagram.
   (c) Classify joints with examples. Name any two joint disorders.
   (d) Write structure and functions of synovial joint with examples.
4. (a) Name the different types of blood groups. Write the importance of blood group.
   (b) Write the composition and functions of blood.
   (c) Write note on disorders of blood.
5. (a) What is RH factor? Write in brief about its importance and incompatibility during blood transfusion.
   (b) Describe the different types of leucocytes and give their functions.
   (c) Write a short note on spleen.

6. (a) Write a neat labeled diagram of heart.
   (b) What is blood pressure? Explain briefly a method used to record it.
   (c) Define hypertension, anginapectoris, myopia and diabetes mellitus.
   (d) Write a short note on blood pressure.
7. (a) Explain the factors affecting blood pressure.
   (b) Explain the anatomy of the heart with the help of labeled diagram.
   (c) Describe in detail the "Cardiac cycle".
8. (a) Explain with neat labeled diagram of respiratory system.
   (b) Explain mechanism of respiration.
   (c) Describe the physiology of respiration.
9. (a) With a neat labeled diagram explain the anatomy of kidney.
   (b) Write short note on nephron and urine formation.
   (c) Explain the physiology of micturition.
   (d) Write the physiology of skeletal muscle contraction in brief.
   (e) Explain reflex arc.
   (f) Write a note on CSF.
10. (a) Explain the functions of cerebrum.
    (b) Draw a neat labeled diagram of brain. Write the functions of cerebrum and medulla oblongata. Draw a reflex arc.
    (c) Draw a neat labeled diagram showing the parts of 'Brain'.
11. (a) Name the different parts of ear. Write the functions of ear.
    (b) Write neat labeled diagram of human eye. What is cataract?
    (c) Write a neat labeled diagram of eye and write the physiology of vision.
12. (a) Draw a neat labeled diagram of ear, explain mechanism of hearing.
    (b) Name the different layers of skin and write the functions of skin.
13. (a) Explain with neat labeled diagram of digestive system.
    (b) Name the enzymes of pancreatic juice and write their uses.
    (c) Name the parts of stomach and list the functions of gastric juice.

14. (a) Define basal metabolism and explain in brief the digestion of carbohydrates.
    (b) Write the role of small intestine in digestive system and absorption of food. List the enzymes in intestinal juice and their functions.
    (c) Name the different parts of G.IT. Enumerate the functions of stomach. Explain the digestion of proteins and fats.
15. (a) Classify vitamins and write in brief the disease caused by deficiency of vit. A and B.
    (b) Name the hormones of adrenal gland and write their functions.
    (c) Name the different endocrine glands. Write the functions of thyroid hormones.
    (d) Name the hormones produced by posterior pituitary gland and give its functions.
16. (a) List the hormones secreted by adrenal cortex of adrenal gland and write important physiological actions of glucocorticoids.
    (b) Write briefly on myxoedema.
    (c) Explain the following terms.
        (i) Endocrine gland
        (ii) Tidal volume
        (iii) Polycythemiavera
        (iv) Cretinism.
    (d) Different between endocrine and exocrine glands. Name the hormones secreted by pancreas. Write their functions in detail.
17. (a) Draw and label the diagram showing internal genital organs in female.
    (b) Define: (i) Puberty (ii) Menopause
    (c) With the help of a neat labeled diagram explain the structure of a sperm.
18. (a) Write the structure and functions of testis.
    (b) Write the effects of sympathetic nervous system on different organs.
    (c) Write short note on menstrual cycle.

12

HEALTH EDUCATION AND COMMUNITY PHARMACY

1. (i) Define the following terms
   (a) Health (b) Disease (c) Health indicators
   (d) Morbidity (e) Mortality (f) Physical health
   (g) Mental health (h) Spiritual health

   (ii) Explain briefly the followings
   (a) Different levels of prevention of disease.
   (b) Factors affecting health.
   (c) Types of health.
   (d) Various indicators of health.
   (e) Determinants of health.
2. What are vitamins? Classify with examples, write a note on the sources, functions, biological role and deficiency of the following vitamins.
   (a) Vit. A (b) Vit. D (c) Vit. B_{12} (d) Ascorbic acid
3. What are proteins? Write a note on types, functions, sources, metabolism and body requirement of proteins?
4. What are minerals? Add a brief note on following minerals.
   (a) Calcium (b) Iron (c) Iodine
5. Write briefly about the following:
   (a) Types of nutrition required for good health.
   (b) Oral rehydration therapy.
   (c) Balance diet.
   (d) Protein energy malnutrition.

6. (i) What are contraceptives, classify, explain the following methods of contraceptives
   (a) Oral contraceptives
   (b) Permanent method of contraception
   (c) Chemical methods of contraception.

   (ii) What is demography and explain demographic cycle?
7. What is family planning, classify and explain different methods of FP and write the role of pharmacist in family planning?
8. What is first aid and explain the first aid treatment of the following?
   (a) Snake bite (b) Shock (c) Fracture (d) Burns
   (e) General treatment of poisoning(f) Food poisoning.
9. (i) Define bacteria, explain the morphology of bacteria with the help of neat labeled diagram.

   (ii) Classify the microbes in various different basis.
10. (i) Explain the isolation of bacteria and various techniques involved in staining of bacteria.

    (ii) Name and explain the diseases spread by house fly, mosquito, rat flea, cattle and dogs.
11. (i) Define immunity, classify, explain the different types of immunity and write difference between active and passive immunity. Add a note on immunization schedule.

    (ii) Classify the modes of transmission of disease with examples.
12. (i) Define epidemiology. Methods of epidemiological studies and methods used to describe disease patterns.

    (ii) Classify immunizing agents with examples and add a brief note on vaccine.
13. Define noncommunicable diseases explain in detail the cause, prevention and control of the following diseases.
    (a) Cancer (b) Diabetes mellitus (c) Blindness
14. (i) Explain the sources of water, supply, pollution, purification of water and add a brief note on methods of "Chlorination".

    (ii) Write briefly about the sound and noise pollution.

15. (i) Give the procedures for the disinfection of feaces, sputum, surgical instruments and linen.
    (ii) Explain the following
    (a) Different types of sanitary wells.
    (b) Different methods of disposal of refuse.
    (c) Disposal of solid waste.

16. Define communicable disease and write the causative agent, incubation period, mode of transmission, prevention and control, treatment of the following diseases.
    (a) Cholera (b) Diphtheria (c) Typhoid
    (d) Malaria (e) Plague (f) Tuberculosis
    (g) Leprosy (h) Amoebiasis (i) Tetanus.

17. What are veneral diseases? Add a brief note on spread, prevention and control of following veneral diseases.
    (a) AIDS (b) Gonorrhea (c) Syphilis

18. Write the brief note on the following.
    (a) Different modes of transmission of diseases.
    (b) Arthropod borne disease.
    (c) Prevention and control of communicable disease.
    (d) Air born diseases.
    (e) Transmission and prevention of intestinal infections.

Section C

QUESTION BANK

(Selected Questions of Paper-Setters' Choice)

13

QUESTION BANK

BIOCHEMISTRY AND CLINICAL PATHOLOGY

1. Proteins and their Biological Role

1. Write a note on essential amino acids.
2. Write any two tests of identify proteins.
3. Write a note on
   (a) Kwashiorkor (b) Marasmus.
4. Discuss the biological functions of proteins.
5. What are amino acids? Discuss their biological functions.
6. What are essential amino acids? Name six essential amino acids.
7. Write a note on denaturation of proteins?
8. Define proteins? Classify with examples.
9. Write biological value of proteins.
10. Classify simple and conjugated proteins with examples.
11. Give the chemical equation involved in the ninhydrin test.
12. Write a note on colour reactions of proteins.
13. Discuss the acid-base behaviour of amino acids.
14. Enumerate the various roles played by proteins.

2. Carbohydrates

1. What are carbohydrates? Classify them with examples.
2. Describe the one test for each of the following
   (a) Reducing sugar (b) Non-reducing sugar
   (c) Ketone sugar (d) Starch
3. Describe nutritional functions of carbohydrates.

4. What are disaccharides? Write the structure of maltose and give a test to distinguish it from sucrose.
5. Write any two tests to identify carbohydrates.
6. Write the chemical equation of Benedict's test.
7. Define reducing and non-reducing sugar.
8. Write the one test used to distinguish them.
9. Write the structure of glucose and fructose and give one test differentiate them.
10. Explain following tests to detect carbohydrates giving its principles.
    (a) Molish test (b) Osozone test
11. Write briefly glycogen storage diseases.
12. Write a note on muta rotation.

3. Lipids

1. Define the following terms
   (a) Iodine number (b) Saponification number
   (c) Acid number (d) Acetyl number
2. Define lipids. Classify them with examples.
3. Write a note on biological role of lipids?
4. What is the importance of unsaturated fatty acids? Write the names and structures of any three unsaturated fatty acids.
5. What are fatty acids? How they are classified? Write the qualitative test for lipids.
6. What is the principle and procedures involved in the estimation of cholestrol?
7. Write a note on atherosclerosis.
8. Define oils and fats and discuss hydrolysis and transification of oils.
9. Write a note on fatty acids? What are their biological functions. Write a note on essential fatty acids.

4. Vitamins and Coenzymes

Section A

1. Name two co-enzymes and give their biological functions.
2. Classify vitamins and name the disease called by the deficiency of each vitamins.

3. Explain the biological functions of vitamin and vitamin K.
4. Give the functions and deficiency of vitamin D and vitamin K.
5. Write briefly pellegra and beriberi diseases.
6. List out the important functions of vitamin C.
7. Give the structure biochemical role of pyridoxine.
8. Give a biological role, source daily requirements and deficiency conditions of thiamine.
9. What are the functions of vitamin C and its deficiency disease?
10. What are co-factors and co-enzymes? Give examples.
11. Classify vitamins with examples.
12. Give the structure and functions of thamine pyrophosphate.

Section B

1. Give the sources, chemistry, biochemical functions deficiency and daily requirements of vitamin A.
2. (a) What are vitamins, write water soluble vitamins?
   (b) Write the structure, sources daily requirements functions and deficiency symptoms of vitamin D.
   (c) Write a note on fat soluble vitamins.
3. Write a note on co-enzymes.

5. Water and Mineral Metabolism

1. Explain the role of water in life process.
2. Write a note on functions of iron and copper in the body.
3. Describe the physiological role of copper and iron.
4. Write biological functions of phosphate.
5. Give the biological role of calcium and phosphorous in the body.
6. Enumerate the role played by iron and sodium in the body.
7. Write short notes on water balance of the body.
8. Explain the role of water and minerals in the life process.

6. Enzymes

Section A

1. Name any two co-enzymes and give their biological functions.
2. Explain allostirine enzyme inhibition.

3. Discuss the effect of pH and temperature on enzyme activity.
4. Write a note on the specificity of enzymes.
5. Discuss the effects of substrate and enzyme concentration on the enzyme catalyzed reactions.
6. Enumerate some enzymes preparations used in medicine and pharmacy giving their source and specific applications.
7. What are the factors affecting enzyme actions? Explain with examples.
8. Give details about enzymes of pharmaceutical importance.

Section B

1. (a) Discuss IUB classification of enzymes.
   (b) Describe briefly special properties of enzymes.
   (c) Write a note on competitive enzyme in inhibition.
2. (a) What are enzymes? Classify them with examples.
   (b) What are co-enzymes write any co-enzymes along with their biological role?
   (c) Give examples of a few enzymes used in therapy along with their specific applications.
   (d) Explain the mechanism of enzyme action.

7. Metabolism

Section A

1. Describe the metabolism of phenylalanines and tyrosine?
2. Describe in brief ketogenesis.
3. Give the significance of HMPS pathways?
4. Discuss the causes and effects of ketosis.
5. Outline the conversion of pyrovate to acetyl co-enzyme A. Write a note on pyruvate dehydrogenase complex.
6. Briefly describe glycogenesis.
7. Write a note on ketone bodies and its functions.
8. What is transamination reaction and explain with examples?
9. Define glucogenesis mention its significance.
10. Explain briefly ketogenesis and ketosis.

11. Discuss the glucose tolerance test.
12. Write a note on hexose monophosphate shunt.
13. What is ketonuria? Explain its significance.

Section B

1. (a) Discuss detail reactions of citric acid cycle and its significance and energetic formed.
   (b) Outline the conversion of pyruvate to acetyl CoA.
2. What is glycolysis? Write the help if flow chart show the reactions of glycolysis giving energetics under aerobic and anaerobic conditions.
3. Give on account of B oxidation of palmitic acid. Give its significance and energetics.
4. (a) Explain glycogenolysis occur in the liver along with its significance.
   (b) What is gluconeogenesis? What is its importance write the distinctive reactions of gluconeogenesis?
5. (a) Discuss in detail hexose monophosphate shunt pathway? Give its significance.
   (b) Gluconeogenesis.
6. (a) Describe the metabolism of phenyllalanine and tyrosine.
   (b) Explain decorboxilation with examples.
   (c) Describe the catabolism of phenyllalanine and tyrosine.
7. Explain transamination, de-amination, de-carboxylation of amino acids with one examples for each. What is significance of each of these reactions.
8. Discuss anaerobic oxidation of glucose. Write a note on ascorbic acid.
9. (a) Explain the mechanism by which nitrogenous waste is eliminated from the body.
   (b) Write a note on functions of cholestrol in the body.
10. (a) Define glycolysis briefly discuss the process of glycolysis. Write a note on its significance.
    (b) Briefly indicate the conditions that may lead to diabetes mellitus. What are its symptoms how is it generally related.

11. Discuss in detail reactions of krebs citric acid cycle. Write about the significance and its energetics. Explain de-corboxilation of amino acids with examples.

8. Pathology of Blood and Urine

Section A

1. Name the ketone bodies and bile pigments. How do you identify them in urine?
2. What are lymphocytes? Give their significance in health and disease.
3. Write the principle involved in the test for ketones bodies and the salts?
4. Write four abnormal constituents of urine and their significance.
5. Explain the role of platelets in health and disease.
6. Discuss the pathological conditions in which the glucose and ketone bodies appear in urine? Write one test to detect them in urine.
7. How creatinine is syntheses in the body? Give one test for the presence of creatinine.
8. Explain the role lympocytes in diseases.
9. Name the bile salts and bile pigments? How do you identify them in urine?
10. Give the test for sugar, and ketone bodies in the urine and write about their clinical significance.
11. What are lympocytes? Discuss their role in the body.
12. What is significance creatinine in the body? How is it formed?
13. Write note on diabetes mellitus.
14. What are platelets? What is their role in the body?

Section B

1. (a) Discuss in detail about the abnormal constituents at urine and their significance in diseases.
   (b) What are lympocytes? Give their significance in health and disease.
2. What is urea? Where is it produced? Write the specific test to identify urea in urine.

3. Name the abnormal constituents of urine. How are they tested? What is the significance at each of these tests.
4. (a) Discuss in detail about the abnormal constituents of urine and their significance in diseases.
   (b) Discuss the role of lympocytes in health.
5. (a) What are the normal constituents at blood and give their significance?
   (b) What are abnormal constituents at urine? How these are detected in the laboratory?

HUMAN ANATOMY AND PHYSIOLOGY

1. Introduction

Section A

1. Define the terms anatomy and physiology.
2. Define the following terms.
   (a) Physiology (b) Histology
   (c) Health (d) Splanchology

2. Cell

1. Define cell and name the different organelles of cell.
2. Write the structure and function of mitochondria.
3. Write short note on mitochondria.

3. The Tissues

Section A

1. Classify muscular tissue and write the characteristic feature of any one of them.
2. Define tissues, classify them.
3. Define tissue. Name different types of connective muscular tissues.
4. Classify tissues.
5. Name the different types of muscle tissue. Discuss the skeletal muscle.
6. Define tissue. The different types connective and muscular tissues.
7. Write the differences between the properties of skeletal muscular and cardia muscle.

8. Classify tissues with an example for each class. Write the functions of spithelial tissues.

Section B

1. (a) Describe the various types of connective tissue with example.
   (b) Name the different types of teeth and give the structure of tooth.

4. Organs and Systems

5. The Skeletal System

Section A

1. Name the bones of lower limb.
2. Define bone, classify bones with examples.
3. Name of the bones of skull.
4. Name the following.
   (i) The only movable bone of the face.
   (ii) Hormones of posterior pituitatry gland.
   (iii) The mixed gland (exo- and endocrine gland).
   (iv) The space between the lungs.
   (v) Hardesh connective tissue.
   (vi) The disease caused by the virus ELISA-HIV.
   (vii) The disease caused by deficiency of clotting factor VIII.
   (viii) Intravascular clotting of blood.
5. List the functions of bone.
6. Explain the identifying features scapula with a neat labeled diagram.

Section B

6. Joints of the Skeleton

Section A

1. Explain synovial joint with a diagram.
2. Name the bones of upper limb. Classify joints.
3. Classify joints with examples. Name any two joint disorders.
4. Write structure and functions of synovial joint with examples.

5. Name the bones of upper limb and give their locations in the body.
6. Explain synovial joint with diagram.
7. Write short note on rheumetoid arthritis.

Section B

7. Blood

Section A

1. Name the different types of blood groups. Write the importance of blood groups during blood transfusion.
2. Write the composition and functions of blood.
3. Classify WBCs and write their functions.
4. Write the composition and functions of blood.
5. Name the blood groups—write the importance of RH system.
6. Briefly write about RBC.
7. Write note on disorders of blood.
8. Define ESR, what is its importance?
9. What is RH group? Write it significance.
10. Write the composition and functions of plasma.
11. Explain the mechanism of clotting of blood.
12. Explain ESR and give to significance.
13. Define ESR and its importance.
14. What is RH factor? Write in brief about its importance. And incompatibility during blood transfusion.
15. List out the organic constituents of plasma.
16. Write brief note on incompetability of blood groups.
17. Write a brief note on erythropoiesis.

Section B

1. Write the composition and functions of blood. What is blood clotting? Explain the mechanism of clotting in detail.
2. (a) Describe the development, structure and functions of erythrocytes and give its normal count.

   (b) Write the structure and functions of tests.

3. (a) Describe the different types of leucocytes and give their functions.
4. (a) What is RH factor? Mention its clinical importance.
   (b) Classify leucocytes, mention their normal values and functions.
   (c) Add a note on origin, fate, normal values and functions of haemoglobin.
5. Explain erythropoesis.
6. Describe the morphology of leucocytes and mention their respective functions.

8. Lymphatic System

Section A

1. Give the structure and functions of spleen.
2. Write short note on spleen.

Section B

9. Cardiovascular System

Section A

1. Write a neat labeled diagram of heart.
2. Explain in brief systemic and pulmonary circulation.
3. What is ECG? Describe the components of normal ECG in lead I.
4. What is hypertension? Write regulatory mechanisms of blood pressure.
5. What is blood pressure? Explain briefly a method used to record it.
6. Define the following terms.
   (a) Hypertension (b) Anaemia (c) Cardiac arrthmia.
7. Write a brief account of portal circulation of blood.
8. Define blood pressure and name the factors regulating blood pressure.
9. Add a note on junctional tissues of heart.
10. Define hypertension, anginapectoris, myopia and diabetes mellitus.

11. Define cardiac cycle. Name the events and mention their durations.
12. Describe the normal ECG with a diagram and mention kits clinical importance.
13. Add a note on special functional tissues of the heart.
14. Write a short note on blood pressure.
15. Explain the factors affecting blood pressure.

Section B

1. Name the special functional tissues of the heart and write their functions. Explain the changes taking place in the heart during one heart beat in detail.
2. Write the functions of cardiovascular system. Write the physiology of heart. Name the different values and their locations.
3. Explain the anatomy of the heart with the help of labeled diagram and explain the cardiac cycle.
4. With the help of neat labeled diagram explain the cardiac cycle anatomy and physiology of heart. Name the special junctional tissues.
5. (a) Describe in detail the "Cardian cycle".
   (b) Explain the following terms
   (i) Cardiac output (ii) ECG
6. (a) With a neat labeled diagram describe the internal structure of heart.
   (b) Explain heart sounds and give their significance.
7. (a) Draw a neat labeled diagram of heart showing its internal structure.
   (b) Explain how the blood circulates through the heart and lungs.
8. (a) Describe the events taking place during a cardiac cycle.
   (b) What are the factors which hasten coagulation of blood?
9. With the help of a neat labeled diagram describe the anatomy of heart and explain cadiac cycle.

10. Respiratory System

Section A

1. Explain in short internal and external respiration.
2. With a neat labeled diagram, explain the anatomy of lungs.

3. Write a neat labeled diagram of respiratory system.
4. Explain in short internal and external respiration.
5. Explain mechanism of respiration.
6. Give the structure and functions of harynx.
7. Write briefly on internal respiration.
8. Explain the mechanism of internal respiration.

Section B

1. Write a neat labeled diagrm of respiratory system. Describe the mechanism of respiration. Name the different regulatory centres of respiration.
2. (a) Describe the physiology of respiration.
   (b) Discuss the structure and functions of liver.
3. Name all the respiratory muscles and explain the process of inspiration.
4. Name the respiratory muscles and explain the mechanism of respiration.

11. Urinary System

Section A

1. Explain the physiology of micturation.
2. With a neat labeled diagram explain the anatomy of kidney.
3. What is a nephron? Write a neat labeled diagram of nephron.
4. Write a neat labeled diagram of urinary system.
5. Write a neat labeled figure of nephron.
6. Explain the physiology of micturition.
7. Explain micturation and defecation.
8. Write the abnormal constituents of urine.
9. Describe the anatomy of kidney.

Section B

1. Describe the structures and functions of nephron, explain the mechanism of urine formation.
2. (a) Describe the structure and functions of nephron.
   (b) Explain the chemical digestion food in small intestine.

3. Explain the processes by which the urine is formed.
4. (a) With a neat labeled diagram of nephron, describe its structures and explain the formulation of urine.
   (b) Write two important physiological functions of
   (i) Adipose tissue (ii) Haemoglobin
   (iii) Oestrogen (iv) Growth harmone.
5. Write a neat labeled diagram of nephron and explain the mechanism of formation of urine. Name the normal constituents of urine.

12. The Muscular System

Section A

1. Write the physiology of skeletal muscle contraction in brief.
2. Describe the physiology of neuromuscular function.

Section B

13. The Physiology of Muscle

Section A

1. Write the physiology of muscle contraction.

Section B

1. Explain the physiology of muscle contraction. Name the different types of vertebrae. Explain the terms anaemia and myopia.
2. Explain the physiology of contraction of skeletal muscle.
3. Write the functions of cerebellum.
4. Write the composition and function of cerebrospinal fluid.
5. Explain reflex are.
6. Explain myelinated neurone with a diagram.
7. Describe the structure of neuron with a neat labeled diagram.
8. Write a note on CSF.
9. Explain the functions of cerebrum.

Section B

1. Draw a neat labeled diagram of brain. Write the functions of cerebrum and medulla oblongata. Draw a reflex are.
2. Write a neat labeled diagram of brain. Write the functions of cerebrum and hypothalamus.

3. Write the effects of sympathetic nervous system on different organs. Write the functions of cerebellum and hypothalamus.
4. (a) Draw a neat labeled diagram showing the parts of brain.
   (b) Write the functions of cerebrum and cerebellum.
5. With the help of a labeled diagram describe the various parts of 'Brain'
   (a) Mention the important of insulin describe the anatomy of brain.
   (b) Write a note on insulin and its regulation.
6. With a labeled diagram describe the anatomy of brain.
   (a) Give brief account of disorders of thyroid gland.
7. (a) Draw the diagram of CNS and add a note on cerebrum.
   (b) Explain sympathetic and parasympthatetic nervous system and compare their actions on various organs.
8. Define reflex action and differentiate between central nervous system and autonomick nervous system.
9. (a) Define reflex action. Draw the diagram of reflex are.
   (b) Enumerate the functions of parasympathetic system on CNS.
   (c) Write short note on meninges.

14. Autonomic Nervous System

Section A

1. Write the effects of sympathetic nervous system on different organs.
2. Name the organs innervated by autonomic nervous system.
3. Describe reflex are with the help of diagram.

Section B

1. (a) Briefly explain ANS.
   (b) Add a note on general circulation.

15. Organs of Special Senses

Section A

1. Name the different parts of ear, with the functions of ear.
2. What are the rods and cones? Write their functions.
3. Explain the mechanisms of vision.

4. Name the errors of refraction in the eye and give its remedies.
5. Define the terms amenorrhoea, glaucoma, anaemia and graves disease.
6. Write neat labeled diagram of human eye, what is cataract?

Section B

1. Write a neat labeled diagram or ear. Explain the physiology of hearing and impaired hearing.
2. Write a neat labeled diagram of eye and write the physiology of vision.
3. Write a neat labeled diagram of ear. Write the physiology of hearing.
4. Draw a neat labeled diagram of Eye. Explain the physiology of vision. What is glaucoma?
5. Draw a neat labeled diagram of ear, explain mechanism of hearing.
6. (a) With a neat labeled digram discuss the parts of human Eye.
   (b) Name the different types of vertebrae and explain the functions of bone.
7. Discuss the structure of eye. Write briefly the errors of refraction.
8. Draw a neat labeled diagram of human ear and explain the mechanism of hearing of sound.
9. With the help of a neat labeled diagram of eye explain the mechanism of vision and add a note on glaucoma.

16. Skin and Regulation of Body

Section A

1. Name the different layers of skin and write the functions of skin.
2. Write the different functions of skin.
3. Draw a neat labeled diagram of the skin.
4. Explain the skin regulates the body temperature.
5. Enumerate the functions of skin.

Section B

1. Describe the structure and functions of skin.

17. Digestive System

Section A

1. Write a neat labeled diagram of digestive system.
2. Write the physiology of defecation.
3. Name the enzymes of pancreatic juice and write their uses.
4. List the enzymes of digestive system.
5. Name of the parts of stomach and list the functions of gastric juice.
6. Enumerate the functions of saliva.
7. Define basal metabolism and explain in brief the digestion of carbohydrates.
8. Name the parts of stomach. List the functions stomach.
9. Draw a labeled diagram of tongue. Name the functions of tongue.

Section B

1. Draw a neat labeled diagram of GIT. Explain the digestion and absorption of carbohydrates in GIT. Listing out the enzymes involved in it.
2. Write the role of small intestine in digestive system and absorption of foood. List the enzymes in intestinal juice and their functions.
3. Name the different parts of GIT. Enumerate the functions of stomach. Explain the digestion of proteins and fats.
4. Name the various parts of digestive system. Write the physiology of digestion and absorption in small intestine.
5. (a) Discuss the digestion of food in small intestine.
   (b) Explain the formation of urine.
6. Explain the physiology of digestion proteins.
7. Explain in detail with neat labeled diagram the structure and functions of stomach.
8. (a) Explain the process of digestion of carbohydrates.
   (b) List the functions of large intestine.
9. Describe the functions of pancreas.

18. Accessory Organs of Digestion

Section A

1. Write the composition of pancreatic juice and their functions.

2. Write the structure and functions of liver.
3. Name the functions of liver.
4. Write the functions of liver.
5. Write the exercise and endocrine functions of pancreas.
6. Name of enzymes of pancreatic juice and write their functions.

Section B

1. With the help of neat labeled diagram describe the anatomy of liver and explain its functions.

Section A

1. Classify vitamins and write in brief the diseases caused by deficiency of
   (a) Vitamin D (b) Vitamin B_{12}

Section B

19. Endocrine System

Section A

1. Define endocrine glands. Name the harmones of anterior pituitary gland and write their functions.
2. Name the hormones of adrenal gland and write their functions.
3. Write the functions of hypothalamus.
4. Name the different endocrine glands. Write the functions of thyroid hormones.
5. Give the functions of thyroid hormone.
6. Name the harmones of the thyroid glands, write the functions of thyroxine.
7. Give a brief account of disorders of thyroid gland.
8. Name the hormones produced by posterior pituitary gland and give its functions.
9. Name the endocrine glands. Mention the hormones of posterior pituitary and their functions.
10. List the hormones secreted by adrenal cortex of adrenal gland and write any two important physiological actions of gluco-corticoids.
11. Write briefly on myxedema.

12. Write briefly on posterior pituitary gland.
13. Explain the following terms.
    (a) Endocrine gland (b) Tidal volume
    (c) Polycythemiavera (d) Cretinism

Section B

1. Differentiate between endocrine and exocrine glands. Name the hormones secreted by pancreas. Write their functions in detail.
2. With labeled diagram, describe the structure and functions of thyroid gland.
3. Enumerate the functions of platelets and give its importance.

20. Reproductive System

Section A

1. Write the structure and functions of testis.
2. Write a neat labeled diagram of female reproductive system.
3. Write a short note on menstrual cycle.
4. Write a short note about menstrual cycle.
5. Write a note on menstrual cycle.
6. Write a note on oral contraceptives.
7. Add a note on puberty in females.
8. Name the female sex hormones. What are their functions?
9. Write short note on menstrual cycle.

Section B

1. (a) Name the accessory organs of digestion discuss pancreas.
   (b) Draw a neat labeled diagram of internal reproductive organs of female, explain ovary.
2. Draw and label the diagram showing internal genital organs in female.
3. Draw a neat labeled diagram of female reproductive system.
4. Define the following
   (a) Puberty (b) Menopause.

21. Process Reproduction

Section A

1. With the help of a diagram explain the structure of a sperm.

PHARMACOGNOSY

Chemical Test

Section A

1. Give the chemical tests for identification of the following
   (a) Isapaghulu (b) Pale catechu
   (c) Benzoin (d) Asafoetida
2. Give two tests to identify aloes.
3. Explain the following tests.
   (a) Combined umbelliferone tests
   (b) Fiche's test
4. Give one chemical test for identification of the following
   (a) Honey (b) Agar
   (c) Cinnaman (d) Benzoin
5. Mention any 2 specific chemical tests for the identification of the following
   (a) Agar (b) Asafoetida (c) Aloe
   (d) Catechu (e) Acacia
6. Describe the following tests
   (a) Combined umbelliferone test
   (b) Hayer's test.

Section B

1. Write the chemical tests useful in the identification of the following
   (a) Agar (b) Gelatin
   (c) Benzoin (d) Honey
2. Write a note on Borntragor's and modified Borntragor's test.

MORPHOLOGICAL MICROSCOPY CHARACTERS

Section A

1. Describe the morphological characters of clove and ipecac.
2. Describe the morphological characters of
   (a) Vasaka (b) Clove

3. Describe the morphological characters with an eat labeled diagram for:

   (a) Nux vomica (b) Fennel

4. Describe the morphological features of umbelliferous fruits.
5. With a neat labeled diagram describe microscopical characters of the following drugs.

   (a) Senna leaf (b) Fennel

6. Give macroscopical characters with source and uses.

   (a) Clove (b) Digitalis leaf

7. Write the morphological characters of fennel and ginger.

Section B

1. Give the anatomical characters of the following with the help of a neat labeled diagram.

   (a) Fennel (b) Cinchona

2. Write a note on opium.
3. With the help of a neat labelled diagram describe microscopy of

   (a) Clove (b) Cinnamon

4. Write a neat labeled diagram and explain the anatomical characters of senna.
5. Mention any one crude drug belonging to the family Solanaceae. Give its BS. Explain its morphological features.
6. With the help of a neat labeled diagram, describe the anatomical characters of

   (a) Nux vomica (b) Clove

7. Give the anatomical charater of the following with the help of a neat labeled diagram.

   (a) Ginger.

Introduction

Section A

1. Define

   (a) Stomatal index (b) Pharmaceutical aids.

2. What is the difference between organized and unorganized drugs. Give examples.

Section B

1. Write note on antiseptics and disinfectant.
2. What are different types of evaluation. Explain the physical method of evaluation.
3. Define evaluation? Name different methods of evaluation. Discuss morphological and microscopical evaluation with suitable examples.
4. Discuss in detail about evaluation of crude drugs.
5. Write a note on chemical evaluation of crude drugs.

Crude Drugs

Section A

1. What are official source, family, c.c. of tragacantha and nutmeg.
2. Give the official source and uses of drugs containing the following c.c.

   (a) Vitamin C (b) Arabin

   (c) Commiphoric acid (d) Myricin
3. Name the drugs belonging to the following classes. Write their botanical source and c.c.

   (a) Antitumour (b) Antirheumatic (c) Antimalarial

   (d) Antitussive (e) Antidysentric (f) Oxytoxic

   (g) Antiseptic
4. Name two drugs containing vitamins along with their source, family, chemical constituents and uses.
5. Give the chemical identification of the following family (one drug)

   (a) Malvaceae (b) Solanaceae

   (c) Ferrulic (d) Reutaceae
6. Give BS and uses of the drugs containing following constituents.

   (a) Vincristine (b) Emetine

   (c) Ferrulic acid (d) Clove
7. Name BS chemical C and uses of Amla and Aloes.
8. Give the name and uses of any one drug belonging to the following families.

(a) Zingiberaceae (b) Cauraccae

(c) Leguminisae (d) Euphorbiaccae

9. Name the important chemical constituents and uses of the following:

(a) Senna (b) Isapgol

(c) Plate catechu (d) Honey

10. Give one example of a drug used as the following.

(a) Colouring agent (b) Insecticide

(c) Emulsifying agent (d) Antigout

11. Give the biological source and therapeutic effect for the following.

(a) Vasaka (b) Colchicum

(c) Vinca (d) Chaulmoogra oil

12. Give the source in which the following constituents are present give their uses.

(a) Eugent (b) Hyoscyamind

(c) Strychine (d) Reserpine

13. Name the important c.c. present in the following drus and mention their uses.

(a) Coriander (b) Cannabis

(c) Clove (d) Gokhru

14. Give the biological source and uses of:

(a) Liquorice root (b) Pyrethrum

15. Give biological source and active principle of any 2 drugs used in perfumery and flavouring.

16. Give the name, official source and uses ofare drug each belonging to following families.

(a) Acanthacea (b) Loganeaceae

(c) Euphorbiaceae (d) Myrtaceae.

17. Mention and carminatives with their official source and family.

18. Name 2 anti-rhematic drugs along with their official source, family and AC.

19. Mention the name, BS family and uses of crude drugs containing.
    (a) Ferulic acid (b) Bassorin
    (c) Invert sugar (d) Cannabinol.
20. Name the source, AC and uses of
    (a) Neem (b) Tobacco (c) Black pepper
    (d) Linseed (e) Amla (f) Shark liver oil
21. Mention source CC and uses for any four:
    (a) Castor oil (b) Pyrethrum (c) Bees-wax
    (d) Clove (e) Gokhru
22. Write OS, and uses of crude drugs containing
    (a) Cannabinol (b) Bassorin (c) Reserpine
    (d) Papain (e) Cantharidin (f) Atropine
    (g) Myrisicin (h) Curcumin
23. Give one example for each of the following and write their uses.
    (à) Rhizome (b) Fungus
    (c) Kernal (d) Leaf
24. Name and give the active constituents and one drug belonging to the following
    (a) Papveraceae (b) Rutaceae
    (c) Umbelliferae (d) Apocynaceae.
25. Distinguish between pale catechu and black catechu.
26. Name a drug which is used as the following along with their source.
    (a) Colouring agent (b) Antimalarial
    (c) Antidiabetic (d) Carminative
27. Name a drug which has the following constituents.
    (a) Strychnine (b) Vitamin C
    (c) Menthol (d) Ricinoliec acid

Section B

1. Write a note on drugs having antiseptic property.

CULTIVATION AND COLLECTION

Section A

1. Give the source, detailed CC uses and storage conditions of Ergot and Digitalis.

Section B

1. Describe the methods of collection and preparation of Opium and Digitalis.
2. Discuss the collection and preparation of
   (a) Ergot (b) Senna
3. Write a method of collection and preparation of the Opium.

Section A

Chemical Constituents

1. What are alkaloids? Give their properties and general tests for their identification.
2. What are volatile oils and fixed oils? Give two examples for each.
3. Name 2 drugs containing anthracene and tropare alkaloids with their botanical source.
4. Write a note on gums and mucilages.
5. Define glycoside.
6. What are alkaloids? Classify them with examples.
7. What are cardiac glycosides? Give their identifications tests.
8. What are volatile oils? How volatile oils are separated by oteam, distillation method.
9. What are enzymes? Explain papaine.
10. Give the example each of oleoresin and balsamic resin. Mention their official source and uses.
11. Give one specific test each for the identification of cardiac and anthraquinone glycosides. Discuss the test.
12. Define
    (a) Alkaloids (b) Lipids
13 Explain with examples
    (a) Tannins (b) Alkaloids (c) Volatile oils
14. Bring out differences between essential oil and fixed oils.
15. Name 2 drugs containing tempenoids and anthracene glycosides with their botanical source.
16. What are resins? Classify them with examples.
17. Write a note on enzyme of plant origin.

Section B

1. Write a note on drugs containing saponin and tannins.
2. What are cardiac glycosides? Give the source and active constituents of any two drugs used a cardiotonics.
3. Write a note on enzymes.
4. Define tannins, classify them with examples. Give them important properties and tests for identification.
5. What are glycosides? Give their properties and classify them with examples.
6. Name the source, chemical constituents and uses of any two saponin glycosides.

Section A

Introduction

1. Define the following

(a) Pharmacognosy	(b) Astringent
(c) Crude drugs	(d) Laxative
(e) Diuretic	(f) Stomatal index
(g) Palisade ration	(h) Mucilage

Section B

1. Pharmaceutical aids.

Classification

Section A

1. Write a note on morphological classification of crude drugs with examples.
2. What are different methods to classify crude drugs? Give suitable examples.
3. Briefly discuss chemical classification.
4. Morphological characters of ginger.

Section B

1. Discuss various types of classification of crude drugs.

History of Pharmacognosy

Section A

1. Discuss briefly the history of pharmacognosy.
2. Write brief note on crude drug monograph.
3. Write a brief note on the development of pharmacognosy.
4. Write briefly on indegenous system of medicine.

Section B

1. Explain the various indigenous system of medicine.

Section A

Sutures and Ligatures

1. Define suture.
2. Write the source, preparation and uses of cotton.
3. Write source and uses of cotton and regenerated fibres.
4. Differentiate sutures and ligatures.
5. Differences between absorbable and non-absorable sutures with examples.
6. Explain surgical dressings.

Section B

1. Write a note on

   (a) Regenerated fibre (b) Natural fibres
2. What are sutures and ligatures, mention the differences between absorbable and non-absorbable sutures with examples. Explain the chemical of sterilization of catgut.
3. Give the source, preparation and identification of cotton and wool.

Adultration

Section A

1. Define adulteration and classify them with suitable examples.

Section B

1. What is adulteration. Write a brief note on different types of adulteration.

PHARMACEUTICS 1

Capsules

Section A

1. Write a note on gelatin capsules.
2. Differentiate between hand and soft capsules.
3. Write a note on microencapsulation.
4. What is a capsule? Differentiate between hand and soft capsules.
5. Give the composition of hand and soft capsule shells.
6. What are capsules? How are they numbered? What is the composition of a capsule shell.
7. Write a note on capsules.
8. What are the advantages of capsules over other dosage forms?
9. Define and classify capsules? Mention the problem caused in capsule filling.

Section B

1. Mention the problems caused in capsule filling.
2. What is gelatin? How are hard gelatin capsule shells prepared and explain with a neat diagram the manufacture of soft gelatin capsules?

Sterilization

Section A

1. Mention the various methods of sterilization. With examples of materials sterilized by them.
2. Give a brief account of radiation sterilization.
3. What is sterlization? Classify various methods of sterilization.
4. Define isotomic solution.
5. Write a note on gaseous sterilization.
6. Write a short note on aseptic techniques.
7. Suggest and explain method of sterilization for surgical dressing and syringes.

Section B

1. Describe the principle and working of an autoclave.

2. What is clinical sterilization? Name and chemicals which are used in this process.
3. Discuss sterilization by ionizing radiation.
4. Explain preparation of water for injection IP.
5. Describe heat sterilization.

Tablets

Section A

1. Write the classification of compressed tablets.
2. Explain the method of slugging in tablet production.
3. Define tablets. What are the ideal characterstics of a tablets?
4. Classify the different types of tablets with examples.
5. What is dry granulation in tablets processing?

Section A

1. Define tablet and classify the different types of tablets with examples. Explain the various tablet adjuvants with suitable examples.
2. Discuss the manufacturing defects in tablets and their rectification.
3. Name the excipients employed in the production of tablets.
4. Discuss the different stages in the production of tablets by moist granulation technique.
5. Explain the disintegration test for compressed tablets.
6. Describe the various stages to be followed during processing of tablets.
7. Discuss the disintegration test for tablets according to IP.
8. Note on coating of tablets.
9. Describe various processing problems which occur in routine production of tablets.
10. Explain the preparation of tablet by wet granulation method.
11. Mention the different standardization tests carried out on compressed tablets.

Weights and Measures

Section A

1. Give the metric equivalents to the following.

   (a) One grain (b) One fluid ounce

   (c) One pound (d) One minim

2. Find the concentration of sodium chloride required to render 1% w/v solution of cocaine hydrochloride isotonic with blood plasma. The freezing point of 1% w/v solution of cocaine HCl is 0.09'C and that of 1% w/v solution of NaCl is – 0.576'C.
3. A pharmacist mixes together 5 kg of powdered opium containing 10% morphine, what is the % w/w strength of morphine in the resulting powder mixture.
4. Shown stepwise calculation involved in the preparation of 600 ml of 60% v/v alcohol from 95% v/v alcohol.
5. Give the equivalent for

   (a) 2 fluid ounces = table spoonful

   (b) 60 minims = ml

   (c) 60 gram = grains

   (d) 1 fluid ounce = ml

6. Classify the different systems of weights and measures followed in pharmacy with suitable examples.

Section B

1. What proportion should 160%, 50%, 30%, 20% dentrose solution be mixed to get 40% solution.

History of Pharmacy

Section A

1. Write briefly on the history of British Pharmacopoeia.
2. What is pharmacopoeia? Explain when was first Indian Pharmacopoeia published.
3. Write briefly history of IP.

Section B

1. Historical development of IP.

Immunity

Section A

1. What is active and passive immunity?
2. Write the method of manufacture of BCG vaccine.

Section B

1. Define and classify immunity with examples. Explain the method of preparation of smallpox vaccine.
2. Give the method of preparation of diphtheria antitoxin.

Packaging

Section A

1. Write a note on plastics as materials for pharmaceutical packing.
2. What are the different types of containers and closures used in pharmacy.
3. Write a note on glass as a material for packing.
4. Write a note on aerosal packing.
5. Give the advantages and disadvantages of glass containers.
6. What are the desired features of containers?
7. Define containers and closures. Mention the type of materials used for making containers.
8. Define fusion, desiccation, ignition and calcination.
9. What are the desired features of containers?

Section B

1. Explain aerosals.
2. What are fusion, desiccation, ignition and calcinations.

Extraction

Section A

1. Write the various methods of extration with examples.
2. What is modified maceration explain with examples?
3. Write a note on antineous that extraction.
4. Write a note on reverse percolation.
5. Differentiate between reserve percolation and repercolation.

6. What is extraction? Discuss the different types of solvents for the extraction of drugs.
7. What are merits and demerits of maceration and percolation?
8. Define and differentiate tinctures and extracts.
9. How is tincture of orange prepared?

Section B

1. Enumerate and define various extraction processes.
2. With the help of a diagram describe the soxhlet extraction of process.
3. Define maceration. With the help of a neat diagram describe in detail the percolation process.
4. With a neat diagram discuss the containers hot extraction process.

Evaporation

Section A

1. Define drying process and classify driers with the help of a neat diagram explain the construction and working of iyophillizers.
2. Film evaporator. Discuss.
3. Explain freeze drying.
4. Describe the physical factors effecting evaporation. Describe an evaporating pan.
5. Define drying and give the importance of drying process for pharmaceutical. Explain the theory of drying.
6. Discuss the construction, working, advantages and disadvantages of evaporator still and stokes still.
7. Define distillation? List out the various types of distillation processes.
8. Explain tray dryer and bacteria proof filters.
9. Explain construction and working of leaf filter.

Filtration

Section A

1. Write a note on filter aids and filter media. Give two important factors to be considered while selecting the filter media.

2. Give the difference between classification and filtration. What are filter aids.
3. What are the various factors affecting filtration?
4. What are filter aids? Explain them with examples.
5. Write a note on sintered glass filters.
6. What is bacterial filters? Explain any one bacterial filters.

Section B

1. With the help of neat diagram explain the construction an working of plate and frame filter press and sintered glass funnel.
2. Discuss the factors influencing the rate of filtration.
3. Discuss the construction and working of a filter press.
4. Describe the construction and working of a frame and plate type filter press.
5. Explain meta filter.
6. Differentiate between filtration and classification.

Size Separation

Section A

1. Mention various methods used for size seperation of powders. Briefly explain them.
2. What as sieves? State official grades of powders.
3. Give the working of a disintegrator.
4. Give the construction and working of cyclone seperator.
5. What is elutriation? Explain.

Section B

1. With the help of a neat diagram explain the construction and working of fluid energy mill.
2. Explain cyclone rseparator.

Size Reduction

Section A

1. Define communication. Explain the various mechanisms by which the comminution equipment works.

2. Give any 4 merits of size reduction in pharmacy.
3. Describe the construction of a fluid energy mill.
4. What is size reduction? State its importance in pharmacy.
5. What is levigation? Explain the process with examples.

Section B

1. With the help of diagram explain ball mill.
2. Explain triple roller mill and hammer mill.

Mixing

Section A

1. What are the factors considered in mixing process?
2. Write note on silverson mixer cum emulsifier.
3. Write a note on homogeniser.
4. What is mixing? Name the various equipment used for mixing solids, liquids and semi-solids products.

Section B

1. With the help of a neat diagram explain the construction and working of homogenizers.
2. Explain planetary mixer.
3. Explain the working of propeller mixers.

Dosage Form

Section A

1. Classify the various dosage forms with examples.
2. Differentiate between efflorescence and deliuescence.
3. Define dosage form. How are they classified?
4. What is bhasma? How it is prepared?
5. Give a brief account of avaleha and bhasma.
6. What are the merits and demerits of solid dosage forms over liquid dosage form?
7. Differentiate between asavas and aristas.
8. Write a short notes on ayurvedic dosage form.

Distilation

Section A

1. Explain the principle involved in steam distillation.
2. Draw a diagram of the apparatus.
3. What is fractional distillation? Explain.
4. What is distillation under reduced pressure? Give its principle.

Section B

1. Explain steam distillation.

Vaccine and Sera

Section A

1. Mention the significance of tonicity in injection formulation.
2. List the difference between vaccine and sera with examples.
3. What are toxoid? What is the difference between antitoxins and anti-serums?
4. Describe the equipment used for production of water for injection.
5. Write short note on sterile water for injection.

PHARMACHEMISTRY I

Chapter: 1 Tharmacopoeia

1. Write a note on the monograph of IP.
2. Explain pharmacopeial monograph.
3. What is the meaning of official compounds?

Chapter: 2 Acids and Bases

1. Define buffers solution? Mention their importance in pharmaceutical preparation.
2. Define the following terms buffers and acids?
3. List out importance of buffer system using in the pharmacy.
4. Write a note on buffers.
5. Name four compounds assayed by neutralization methods along with their uses.
6. Give the chemistry of assay of boric acid.

7. Discuss in short the physiological acid base balance.
8. What are buffers? Explain the mechanism of buffer action with an example. Briefly discuss the role of buffers in pharmacy.
9. Define acid and base according to various concepts.

Chapter: 3 Antioxidants

1. What are antioxidants? Classify with suitable examples.
2. What are antioxidants? Discuss their importance in pharmaceutical industry and give examples.

Chapter: 4 Gastrointestinal Agents

1. List the official compounds of aluminium and magnesium with their chemical formula.
2. Explain principle involved in the assay of sodium chloride. Magnesium sulphate and magnesium trisilicate.
3. Write the formula and category of the bismuth subcarbonate.
4. How to prepare sodium bisulphate and magnesium trisilicate?
5. Write the formula and category of soda ash.
6. List out the official compounds of aluminium and iron. Mention their uses.
7. What are GIT agents? Classify and define various GIT agents.
8. Mention formula and uses of calcium carbonate.
9. Define antacids and their actions and give the compounds name.
10. What are Astrigents? Give examples and discuss the mechanism actions as antimicrobials.
11. Define and classify GIT agents with examples.
12. Explain the method of preparation of aluminium hydroxide jelly.
13. Write the method of preparation properties, medical uses of alum and magnesium sulphate.

Chapter: 5 Topical Agents

1. Give chemical formula and uses of

   (a) Alum (b) Borax (c) Bleeching powder
2. Discuss the principle and reaction involved in the assay of hydrogen paroxide and preparation of ammoniated mercury.

3. Write a note on protectives. Give the method of preparation of bleaching powder yellow mercuric oxide.
4. Write the formula and category of sodium potassium tartrate, borax.
5. Write the storage condition and medicinal uses of the following hydrogen peroxide, potassium citrate and aluminium hydroxide jelly.
6. Write a note on barium meal.
7. Give the reasons for the following
   (a) Glycerol is used in boric acid assay
   (b) Sulphuric acid is used in the assay of hydrogen peroxide.
8. Define the following
   (a) Equivalent weight (b) Chelating agent
   (c) Anticaries agent (d) Astringent
9. Write the formula and category for the following drugs.
   (a) Tartar emetic (b) Calamine
   (c) Ammoniated mercury
10. Write the chemical formula and complete the reactions.
    (a) Lead acetate + hydrogen sulphide
    (b) Magnesium sulphate carbonate
    (c) Ammonium chloride + (formuladehyde) formaldehyde
    (d) Silver nitrate + potassium chromate
11. Why acetic acid is used in the assay of chlorinated lime?
12. Write a note on redox titrations.
13. Name one inorganic medicinal agents for each of the following
    (a) Scabicide (b) Astringent
    (c) Antacid (d) Emetic
14. Define and give one example of each of the following
    (a) Protective
    (b) Antimicrobial agent and adsorbents
15. Give the storage conditions for the following.
    (a) Iodine (b) Silver nitrite
    (c) Hydrogen peroxide (d) Chlorinated lime

16. Mention the formula and uses of
    (a) Bleaching powder (b) Hydrogen peroxide
17. Write a note on topical agents.
18. Complete and balance the following equations.
    (a) $Ce(SO_4) + FeSO_4$ (b) $H_2O_2 + KMnO_4 + H_2SO_4$
19. How test for swelling properties in Bentonite is performed?
20. Give the chemical composition and uses of the following
    (a) Green vitriole (b) Glauber's salt
    (c) Tartar emetic (d) Talc
21. Name one drug used as
    (a) Scabicide (b) Fungicide (c) Sedative
22. Give the chemical composition and uses of the following
    (a) H_2O_2 (b) Copper sulphate (c) Magnesium sulphate
23. Give method of preparation and storage conditions and uses.
    (a) Bleaching powder (b) Boric acid
24. Give the chemical formula and uses of
    (a) Alum (b) Borax
    (c) Bleaching powder (d) Sodium citrate
25. Discuss the principles and reactions involved in the assay of potassium permanganate.
26. What are topical agents? Define various classes of topical agents. Give examples for each class and add notes on their pharmacological actions.
27. Write a short note on assay of acqueous iodine solutions.
28. Define and discuss with examples protective and adsorbents.
29. Define the following terms
    (a) Buffer (b) Expectorant
    (c) Astringent (d) Emetic
30. List the saline cathatics and explain how do they act.
31. What are topical agents? Classify them with examples.
32. Give the stability and storage conditions for H_2O_2 and bleaching powder.
33. Complete and balance the following reactions.
    (a) Iodine + sodium thiosulphate
    (b) Sodium chloride + silver nitrate

34. Write any two inorganic agents used as astringent.
35. Give the reason acetic acid is used in the assay of chlorinated lime.
36. Write a note on topical agents classify them with examples.
37. Write a note gravimetric analysis.

Chapter: 6 Dental Products

1. Explain the terms with one example for each of the following.
   (a) Anticaries agents (b) Dentifrices
2. Write the descriptive notes on the dental products.
3. Explain the terms with one example
   (a) Dental caries.

Chapter: 7 Inhalanps

1. Define inhalants and add a note on a nitrous oxide.
2. Define inhalants. Give examples. Write the storage and labeling conditions for any one of the inhalants.
3. What is inhalants. Name the official inhalants and mention their uses.
4. Explain properties and uses of oxygen and nitrous oxide.
5. Explain the properties and uses of oxygen and carbon dioxide.

Chapter: 8 Respiratory Stimulants

1. Write a note on the respiratory stimulants.
2. Explain principle involved in assay of ammonium chloride.

Chapter: 9 Expectorants and Emetics

1. Write a note on expectorants giving examples from inorganic compounds.
2. Give the reasons formaldehyde is used in the assay of ammonium chloride.
3. Write the assay of ammonium chloride.
4. Give reasons:
   (a) KCNS is used in copper sulphate assay.
   (b) Formaldehyde is used in NH_4 Cl. Assay.
5. Write note on expectorants giving examples from inorganic compounds.

Chapter: 10 Antidotes

1. Write a short notes on antidotes.
2. Discuss the physiological acid-base balance.

Chapter: 11 Electrolytes

1. Give the chemical formula and uses of sodium citrate.
2. Explain principle involved in sodium chloride.
3. Write a note on major intra- and extracellular electrolytes.
4. Explain briefly about the types of radiations emitted by radioactive isotopes mentioning their characterstics.
5. Discuss the method and preparations of potassium chloride.
6. Write a note on oral rehydration salts.
7. Write a note on oral electrolyte therapy.
8. Define electrolyte combination therapy. Name two preparations with their compositions.

Chapter: 12 Official Compounds of Ca, Fe and I_2

1. Describe the method of preparation ferrous gluconate.
2. Give the synonym chemical formula. Uses and storage conditions of acqueous iodine solution.
3. Write the storage conditions and medicinal uses of ferrous sulphate.
4. Describe the method of preparation of iodine from sea weeds.
5. List the official compounds of magnesium and iron. Give their uses.
6. Name official compounds of sodium and calcium with chemical formula and uses.
7. Give the chemical formula properties, and uses of ferrous sulphate and calcium gluconate.
8. Enumerate the official compounds of iron and iodine.

Chapter: 13 Radiopharmaceuticals

1. Write a note on radiopharmaceuticals.
2. Write a note on radiopaque contrast medium.
3. Write a note on GM counter.

4. Write a note on
   (a) Isotopes (b) Radionuclides
   (c) Mass number (d) Biological effects of radiation
5. What are radiopharmaceuticals? Describe the properties of alpha, beta and gamma radiations. Explain the biological effects radiations. Explain with examples the uses, storage and precautions of pharmaceutically important radioisotopes.
6. Describe the types of radiations emitted radioactive isotopes.

Chapter: 14 Quality Control of Drugs and Pharmaceuticals

1. Define quality control and mention its importance in pharmaceutical preparations.
2. Explain the terms quality control and quality assurance.

Chapter: 15 Impurities of Pharmaceuticals

1. Describe the sources of impurities with examples in pharmaceuticals.
2. Discuss the factors to be considered while fixing the limits for impurities in pharmaceuticals.

Chapter: 16 Limit Tests

1. Describe the procedure involved in the sulphate limit test IP.
2. Write the principles involved, reactions and procedure in the following IP. limit test of
   (a) Iron (b) Lead
3. Difference between assay and limit test.
4. Write the principle involved in the limit test for iron.
5. Write a note on sources of errors.
6. Give the reasons for nitric acid is uded in the limit test for chlorides.
7. Give the reasons for hydrochloric acid. Is used for limit test for sulphates.
8. Discuss the principle involved in the limit test for arsenic. With a neat labeled diagram add a note on apparatus used in arsenic limit test.

9. Describe the principle involved specific conditions and reasons for using various reagents in the limit test for iron and lead (IP).
10. Give the examples for limit tests involving.
    (a) Colour comparison(b) Stain comparison(c) Quantitative LT
11. Give reasons:
    (a) Role of Stannous chloride in stannated hydrochloric acid in arsenic limit text.
    (b) Alcohol and H_2SO_4 in barium sulphate reagent.
12. Write short note on apparatus and procedure arsenic limit test.
13. Explain the term 'Limit test' and the principle involved in the chloride limit test.

Chapter: 17 Identification Tests for Cations and Anions

1. Give the identifications tests with chemical reactions for the following ions.
   (a) Calcium (b) Carbonates
2. Give the identification tests with chemical reactions for the following ions.
   (a) Sodium (b) Nitrate
3. Give two identification tests for calcium and chloride.

HEALTH EDUCATION AND COMMUNITY PHARMACY

Chapter 1: Concept of Health and Disease

Section A

1. What are health indicators? Briefly list out types of indicators.
2. Explain 'Mortality indicates' and "Morbidity indicator" of health.
3. Define physical, mental, social and spiritual health.
4. Discuss briefly the different levels of prevention of disease.
5. Discuss the determinants of health.
6. Define disease and explain modes of prevention of disease.
7. Define health and write the factors affecting it.
8. Describe the various indicators of health.
9. Write a note on prevention of diseases.
10. Define the 4 types of health.
11. How can the diseases be prevented.

Section B

1. Define health and write the factors affecting health.

Chapter 2: Nutrition and Health

Section A

1. Define proteins? List their functions. Name the types of proteins.
2. Write the disease caused due to deficiency of calcium and name the harmones regulating it.
3. Write the functions and sources of ascortic acid.
4. Write a note on malnutrition and vitamin D deficiency.
5. Write the functions, biological role, sources and deficiency states of vitamin A.
6. Add a note on protein energy malnutrition.
7. Explain oral rehydration solution.
8. Write a note on the sources and functions of iron and its deficiency.
9. Write a briefly on balance diet.
10. What are the effect of iron deficiency? How can iron deficiency be treated?
11. Write the source, requirement and deficiency symptoms of proteins.
12. Describe the source, functions and deficiencies symptoms for calcium, iodine.
13. Write the functions and sources of ascortric acid.
14. Write the disease due to differences of calcium and name the harmones regulating it.
15. Describe service, deficiency of vit. B_{12}.
16. Classify vitamins with examples and sources.

Section B

1. (a) Describe the sources, functions and deficiencies of vitamin A and D.

   (b) Write a note on oral-rehydration therapy.

(c) What are proteins? Write a note on their functions, sources, metabolism and body requirements?

(d) What are vitamins? Classify, write a note on the sources, functions and deficiency of vitamin A.

(e) What type of nutrition is required for good health.

(f) Write a note on sources, functions and deficiency of vitamin D.

Chapter 3: Demography and Family Planning

Section A

1. What are contraceptives? Give their classification.
2. What is demography and explain demographic cycle?
3. Enumerate the mechanical method of FP in female and write their merits and demerits.
4. Write a note on IUCD.
5. Define FP enumerate the different methods of FP.
6. Write the advantages and disadvantages of oral contraceptives.
7. Name the chemical contraceptives in female and explain its action.
8. Write the role of pharmacist in FP.
9. Discuss the natural FP methods.

Section B

1. Explain the role of pharmacist in implementing family planning programme.
2. What is FP? Classify the temprorary methods of conception and write a note on condom.
3. (a) Discuss about the permanent methods of contraception.

   (b) Write the role of pharmacist in FP.
4. Write a note on chemical methods of contraception.
5. (a) Classify FP methods.

   (b) Describe any two methods of FP in detail.

Chapter 4: First Aid

Section A

1. Briefly explain the first aid treatment for snake bite.

2. Write the first aid treatment of 'Shock'.
3. Write the first aid treatment of snake bite victim.
4. What is shock? Describe the emergency treatment of shock.
5. What are principles of first aid to be given to a person with a simple fracture?
6. How are the burns managed in an emergency?

Section B

1. (a) Describe the causes, effects and first aid treatment of burns.
   (b) Describe the general treatment of poisoning.
   (c) Write a note on food poisoning.

Chapter 5: Environment Health

Section A

1. What are different methods of disposal of refuse? Write a brief note on any one.
2. List the features of the sanitary well.
3. Give procedures for the disinfection of faces, sputum and linen.
4. Write briefly on disposal of solid wastes.
5. Mention the methods of partification work, write a brief note on any one of them.
6. Write the disinfection procedure faces and surgical instrument.
7. Name the effects of norse pollution and write prevensive measures.

Section B

1. (a) Write a note on sound pollution/noise pollution.
   (b) Explain the sources of water supply, pollution and purification of H_2O.
2. (a) Discuss in detail the advantages, principle and methods of 'chlorination'.
   (b) Give the stages by which water is purified on large scale.
3. Name at least 2 diseases spread by housefly, mosquito, rat flea, cattle and dogs.

Chapter 6: Fundamental Principles of Microbiology

Section A

1. (a) Define bacteria, list out the various techniques used for staining bacteria.
   (b) Write a neat labeled diagram of the bacterial cell.
   (c) Explain the morphology of bacteria with the help of neat diagram.
   (d) Classify microbes on their temperature preference.

Section B

1. (a) Name at least 3 diseases spread by housefly, mosquito, rat flea, cattle and dogs.
   (b) Describe the principles involved in the isolation of bacteria.

Chapter 7: Communicable Diseases

Section A

1. Write the causative organisms for the following diseases.
   (a) Cholera (b) Diphtheria (c) Typhoid (d) Malaria
2. Write a note on indirect methods of transmission of diseases.
3. Classify the modes of transmission diseases with examples.
4. Mention the causative organisms for the following diseases.
   (a) Diphtheria (b) AIDS (c) Gonorrhea (d) Malaria
5. Write a note on prophylaxis and treatment of plague.
6. What are venereal diseases? Add a note on spread and prevention of venereal diseases.
7. Enumerate arthropod borne diseases. How they can be controlled?
8. Write the causative organism for the following diseases.
   (a) Malaria (b) Tuberculosis (c) Typhoid (d) Plague

Section B

1. Discuss the different modes of transmission of diseases.
2. Give the causative agent, mode of transmission and prevention and control of tuberculosis.
3. (a) What are communicable diseases? Give examples.

(b) Write the routes of transmission, prevention control of communi-cable diseases.

4. (a) What are communicable diseases? Give examples.
   (b) Discuss about the transmission of air-born diseases.
   (c) Write the causative agent, mode of transmission and prevention of cholera.
5. Give details on causative agents, mode of transmission and prevention of any four intestinal infections.
6. Discuss arthropod born disease and their control.
7. Discuss the causative agents, mode of transmission, prevention and control of "Malaria".
8. Describe the causative organism, mode of transmission, clinical features and preventive measures of typhoid fever.
9. Enumerate the mode of transmission of communicable diseases.
10. Write the methods of prevention and control of 'Plague'.
11. Write the causative organisms for the following diseases.
    (a) Malaria (b) AIDS (c) Tuberculosis
    (d) Cholera (e) Diphtheria (f) Plague
    (g) Leprosy (h) Amoebiasis
12. Explain AIDS and how can it be prevented.
13. How can tetanus be prevented and teated?
14. Write the methods of prevention and control of 'plague'.
15. (a) What are sexually transmitted diseases?
    (b) Describe the causes, prevention and treatment of AIDS.

Chapter 8: Noncommunicable Diseases

Section A

Section B

1. Define noncommunicable diseases? Explain in detail the cause of cancer, their prevention and control.
2. Discuss the occurance, prevention and control of diabetes mellitus.
3. Write the causes, for 'Diabetes mellitus' and give their methods of prevention and control.

4. (a) Mention the causative factor for blindness.
   (b) Discusss the occurance, prevention and control of blindness.
5. Mention any two noncommunicable diseases and methods to control them for any two diseases.
6. Discuss the occurance, prevention and control of diabetes mellitus.
7. Write the causes, for 'Diabetes mellitus and give their methods of prevention and control.

EPIDEMIOLOGY

Section A

1. Define 'Epidemiology' and give its uses.
2. Classify the modes of transmission of diseases with examples.
3. Write a short note on 'Active unity'.
4. Discuss the methods of epidemiological studies.
5. Define immunity, write the differences between active immunity and passive immunity.
6. What are the adverse reactions of vaccination.
7. Classify immunizing agents with examples.
8. Give an account of immunization schedule.
9. How can the diseases be prevented?
10. Define and classify immunity.

Section B

1. (a) What is a virus? Discuss briefly the various methods of their isolation.
   (b) Write a note on vaccines.
2. (a) Explain different types of immunity.
   (b) Discuss the epidemiological methods used to describe disease patterns.

Reader's Notes

Reader's Notes